NAVIGATING
Problem-based learning

From the reviews

'This is a very comprehensive discussion of the elements that contribute to the structure of PBL programs and the learning needs for individuals to be effective participants in these programs. It brings together all of these components into one manuscript, and therefore it is a very good resource for both teachers and learners.'

Associate Professor Raymond Peterson, Director of the Centre for Medical Education, University of Queensland, Australia

'The student point of view, teaching tips and student tips will be invaluable. The author has picked out components of many subject areas, and written about the relevant components in the context of a medical PBL course. This book has really been written as a "one-stop" guide for learning in a medical PBL curriculum.'

Associate Professor Sally Sandover, PBL Curriculum Coordinator, University of Western Australia, Australia

'The author has identified salient features of teaching and learning in higher education. Although he dwells heavily on medical education I am quite sure that the contents would be useful in other areas of university education especially in the life sciences.'

Professor Dr Khatijah Yusoff, Deputy Vice-Chancellor, University Putra Malaysia, Malaysia

'The main focus of PBL is to generate students and graduates who are independent and life-long learners, good communicators and confident problem-solvers. Dr Azer is an expert in PBL with many years of experience in training tutors and facilitators. This book will be the most useful and essential guide for PBL students and tutors.'

Professor Keh-Min Liu, Associate Dean, College of Medicine, Kaohsiung Medical University, Taiwan

'This book is most valuable for understanding PBL. It is not only useful for medical students ... in fact it is also highly recommended to faculty members and beginning PBL tutors.'

Professor Seiji Yamashiro, Professor of General Medicine, the University of Toyama, Japan

NAVIGATING
Problem-based learning

SAMY AZER

MB, BCh, MSc Medicine, MEd (NSW), PhD (Syd), FACG, MPH (NSW)
Professor of Medical Education
Chair of Medical Education, Research and Development Unit
Director, PBL Training Programs
Faculty of Medicine, Universiti Teknologi MARA, Malaysia
Visiting Professor of Medical Education, University of Toyama, Japan
Formerly Senior Lecturer in Medical Education, Faculty of Medicine,
Dentistry and Health Sciences, the University of Melbourne
and the School of Medicine, the University of Sydney

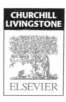

CHURCHILL
LIVINGSTONE
ELSEVIER

Sydney Edinburgh London New York Philadelphia St Louis Toronto

ELSEVIER

Churchill Livingstone
is an imprint of Elsevier

Elsevier Australia
(a division of Reed International Books Australia Pty Ltd)
30–52 Smidmore Street, Marrickville, NSW 2204
ACN 001 002 357

This edition © 2008 Elsevier Australia

Every attempt has been made to trace and acknowledge copyright, but in some cases this may not have been possible. The publisher apologises for any accidental infringement and would welcome any information to redress the situation.

This publication has been carefully reviewed and checked to ensure that the content is as accurate and current as possible at time of publication. We would recommend, however, that the reader verify any procedures, treatments, drug dosages or legal content described in this book. Neither the author, the contributors, nor the publisher assume any liability for injury and/or damage to persons or property arising from any error in or omission from this publication.

National Library of Australia Cataloguing-in-Publication Data

Azer, Samy A.
Navigating problem-based learning.

Bibliography.
Includes index.
ISBN 978 0 7295 3827 5 (pbk.).

1. Problem-based learning - Handbooks, manuals, etc. 2. Study skills - Handbooks, manuals, etc. 3. Group work in education - Handbooks, manuals, etc.
4. Note-taking - Handbooks, manuals, etc. I. Title.

378.17

Publishing Editor: Sophie Kaliniecki
Developmental Editor: Sunalie Silva
Publishing Services Manager: Helena Klijn
Edited by Sybil Kesteven
Proofread by Gabrielle Challis
Illustrations by Joe Lucia
Index by Deirdre Ward
Cover, internal design and typesetting by Jennifer Pace Walter
Printed by Ligare Pty Ltd

FOREWORD

Navigating Problem-Based Learning by Professor Dr Samy Azer is undoubtedly a commendable effort that provides a clear understanding of the problem-based learning (PBL) approach. Over the last twenty years, significant changes have been introduced to teaching and learning in higher education. The current teaching does not aim to load students with factual knowledge and encourage rote learning; rather, it focuses on enhancing students' skills to apply knowledge learnt and enabling them to master problem-solving techniques. It also aims to foster students' analytical and justification skills and motivate them to become life-long learners. These changes in the design of university courses require students to adjust their learning strategies, identify their learning needs, improve their communication skills and foster their collaborative learning. This is particularly important in courses using PBL and giving emphasis to student-centred approaches to learning.

The challenge is that there have, to date, been no resources or books available that cover these skills and enable students to reach their potential. This book covers these needs and adds a useful resource to the library. It provides students with the key skills and tips needed in such courses. Although the book is written mainly for medical and other healthcare students, most chapters are useful to students enrolling in similarly run courses. It covers the different aspects of learning addressed in PBL including: the roles of students in PBL tutorials, keys for successful discussion in tutorials, how to construct good mechanisms, how to identify learning needs, how to improve preparation of learning issues, how to successfully pass examinations, how to manage time effectively and how to deal with stress. The wider application of PBL in today's curricula, beyond the medical and other healthcare professions, makes it imperative that this book be published.

I would like to congratulate the author on his achievement and it is my pleasure to commend this book to you. It reflects the author's expertise in medical education and his devotion to the medical and healthcare professions. I am proud that Professor Azer is an academic in the Faculty of Medicine at Universiti Teknologi MARA, for his worthy contribution to the medical profession indirectly reflects UiTM's achievements. I recommend this book to medical and healthcare students, university educators, course designers and PBL facilitators.

Dato' Seri Professor Dr Ibrahim Abu Shah
Vice-Chancellor
Universiti Teknologi MARA, Malaysia

Contents

Detailed contents

To
My mother
For loving her children and inspiring them into intellectual pursuits

My family
For their support, patience and love

My teachers
For motivating me to ask questions, research, create and construct
new knowledge

My students
For inspiring me to write this book

Preface

People learn in direct proportion to how much fun they are having.
BOB PIKE

I have always asked myself why we are taught *what* to learn yet during my education in Australia and overseas I cannot remember any emphasis given to *how* we learn. This might be the case because I graduated from medicine and the people who taught me were medical graduates rather than educators. But I cannot even remember during my Master of Education—over 13 years ago—any analysis of, or emphasis on this important concept. What I do remember is that during my work on a 2-unit course in educational psychology in 1992, I asked myself how I could turn theories about learning into a recipe that would help students foster their skills. Since then, I have read hundreds of books on education, published a number of research papers on medical education, presented my work at international conferences and contributed to the design of the curriculum in several universities. I have trained over 500 tutors to become problem-based learning (PBL) tutors. The tutors I trained were from a wide range of backgrounds including basic sciences, physiotherapy, nursing, occupational therapy, speech pathology, dentistry, nutrition, health sciences and general practice. I have also trained a number of secondary and primary school teachers to use PBL as an educational tool in the middle years. This broad experience has expanded my interest in education and the process of learning.

Learning is a process that requires understanding of its key elements and continuous practice of its rules. The storage of information in our long-term memory and our ability to retrieve this information and use it in different situations depend to a large extent on the way we learnt that information.

Let me ask you a question. What is your primary goal when you learn? Do you aim to remember just what you have read in a textbook or lecture notes? If that is the case, try this exercise.

Look at the numbers below and try to remember them in their sequence

9, 14, 6, 15, 18, 13, 1, 20, 9, 15, 14

I imagine that some of you might be able to remember all these numbers. But let me ask you: What will be your aim after you have remembered them all? Will you be able to recall them after 2 or 3 hours?

Successful students will ask themselves: Why was I asked to memorise these numbers? What is the value of knowing these numbers? But more importantly, what is the logic behind their sequence?

Some of you might think that these numbers are a code or pin number. This is not the case. What I would like you to do is to think about the rationale for their sequence. Some students who were asked this question looked at mathematical relationships and thought that:

$9 + 14 + 6 = 29$
$15 + 13 + 1 = 29$
$20 + 9 = 29$
$15 + 14 = 29$

But the number 18 was odd and the whole process, although it looks well thought out, cannot explain the rationale for their sequence.

A few students said the number 14 is repeated twice, 15 is repeated twice and 9 is also repeated twice but could not explain why numbers 1, 13, 6 and 20 are not repeated and their significance.

A few students said 9 plus 5 is 14, minus 8 is 6 but it is difficult to find any pattern in this. They also failed to find any relationship when they tried different mathematical approaches.

You might have also attempted all these ways.

Give up? These numbers reflect the sequence of alphabet numbers. A is replaced by 1, B by 2, C by 3 and so on. Can you now work out what these numbers stand for?

This is a simple example. What I would like to emphasise is that your focus should be not on how to memorise information, but rather be on understanding the principles behind it. You might have tried four or five different hypotheses and applied each one to the problem discussed above. What you have tried is a learning process that kept you engaged and triggered your thoughts to understand more about the problem.

During your work on this problem, you might have thought of some questions for me. This is great. Asking good questions helps us to find solutions and learn more about the problem. The students to whom I gave this problem asked me these questions. You might have more questions for me.

- Why are there no numbers higher than 20 in the problem?
- What is the maximum number in your series?
- What do these numbers represent?
- The hypotheses we used were all focused on mathematical rules. We might need to broaden our vision. What should I focus my hypotheses on?

Asking good questions keeps us engaged, helps us deal with uncertainty and uses a scientific approach to solve the problem. More importantly, the aim is not the solution but the learning process behind the problem.

WHY DID I WRITE THIS BOOK?

Worldwide, most medical and healthcare schools have replaced their traditional curriculum and adopted PBL. Learning and teaching in medical and other healthcare professional schools is no longer based on presentation of information. In the PBL approach, teachers are no longer the main source of information; rather, they facilitate discussion. Students work in small groups on a weekly problem; they define their learning issues at the end of the first tutorial then search for the information that can answer their questions. The problem of the week is designed by the faculty and is designed to encourage students to discuss basic and clinical sciences in an integrated way and allow them to discover areas of deficiency in their knowledge.

However, many students find it difficult to change their learning style, work with others in small groups or use the educational opportunities provided in PBL in an effective way. As a senior lecturer in medical education at the University of Sydney and the University of Melbourne, I mentored a number of first- and second-year medical students who were challenged by problem-based learning as a learning style. Here are some of the issues they raised:

> … I do not know what the aim of problem-based learning is. Why did you choose this approach in the new course?

… There is too much to do in the course and I am not always sure if I have studied enough or not. Are there any ways to know?

… How can I improve my performance in PBL tutorials?

… I understand that you train our PBL tutors to enhance their facilitation skills. Why didn't you run student workshops as well on how to become students in a PBL course and what's expected from them?

… I get frustrated with the new role of our PBL tutors and the way they do not like to provide direct answers to our questions. I came from a system were it was the duty of the teacher to answer students' questions. It isn't my job to search for information, it's too time consuming.

… How much detail should we discuss in our PBL tutorials? Are there any ways to enhance our skills as we create our mechanisms?

… While our PBL cases are based on integration of knowledge across disciplines and building links between basic and clinical sciences, I find it very challenging to prepare my learning issues. The problem is, most textbooks are not integrated and collecting information from different textbooks is really a challenge for all of us. Are there ways to deal with this?

These problems are real. In this book I give you a set of tools and strategies to improve your performance in PBL tutorials, enhance your study skills and add new dimensions to what you want to achieve from your course. This book provides you with the keys for success: you will see improvements within 4–5 weeks of using it.
Other reasons for writing the book are:
- There are no books in the market written specifically for PBL medical students to prepare them in a practical way for their course.
- The skills I cover in my book are often not addressed adequately by PBL course designers. Course designers usually present a lecture on the theoretical aspects of PBL, how PBL works and why we need to use PBL. They may train their tutors to facilitate tutorials, but they rarely train their students to understand their role in PBL tutorials, to address the practical aspects of how to adapt their learning styles to meet the objectives of the new curriculum, to provide them with the keys for success in the new curriculum and to master self-directed learning or to prepare for scenario-based questions and the PBL-style questions commonly used in assessment.
- Because of this gap I prepared a paper, 'Becoming a student in a PBL course: twelve tips for successful group discussion' (published in *Medical Teacher*). This paper addresses some of the needs of students in a PBL course in a practical way. Eight or nine universities worldwide recommended my paper to their students and included it in their list of resources: this response triggered the idea for my book.
- Communications from medical students, educators, course designers and deans of medical and healthcare professional schools in Australia, Japan (University of Toyama), Malaysia (Universiti Teknologi and MARA) and Taiwan (Kaohsiung Medical University) provided support for such a book.
- The number of medical schools which have adopted PBL curricula has increased dramatically over the last 15 years. Searching MEDLINE shows that the number of research papers on PBL from these schools has increased from 299 papers in a

20-year period (1975–1995) to 2196 in only a 10-year period (1995–2005)—a more than seven-fold increase in half the time. A significant number of these publications have been submitted from universities that have introduced PBL in the last 15 years.

- The universities where I have been a keynote speaker and visiting scholar (Kaohsiung Medical University, Toyama Medical University and Universiti Teknologi MARA) are in the process of introducing PBL into their curricula and are practical examples of such changes to medical curricula in our region; further argument for the need for such a book.

WHO SHOULD READ IT?

If you are a student in a PBL course, this book is a practical guide for improving your academic performance. It is particularly useful to students at undergraduate and postgraduate levels enrolled in courses in medicine, nursing, physiotherapy, dentistry, occupational therapy, speech pathology, veterinary sciences, basic sciences, teaching, law and forensic examination which use PBL.

This book is also recommended if you are a year 12 high school student or a graduate student interested in studying a medicine/healthcare course with a PBL curriculum. Reading this book a month or two before starting your course will prepare you for the philosophy of the course and show you how you can change your study skills to accommodate the PBL design.

If you are a PBL tutor, a medical/healthcare educator or an educator in any other discipline that uses problem-based learning, this book will provide you with tools to improve your students' performance in PBL tutorials.

This book is also useful to any educator who uses small-group learning and self-directed learning in their teaching and finds it difficult to prepare for the classes. Using this book will ensure successful implementation and better outcomes.

Even if you have been a student in a PBL course for a year or more, you will pick up new skills by reading this book. You will discover dozens of tips and techniques on how to maximise your performance and study skills, including the following:

- Your role in PBL tutorials and how you can improve your input to group discussion.
- How to lead discussion in your group without being dominating or upsetting other members.
- What to do when your group is arguing an issue and the discussion is not progressing.
- What your tutors look for when determining your performance.
- How to express your ideas effectively and share your ideas even if you aren't sure they are valid.
- How to take notes that improve your understanding.
- How to search for new information and prepare your learning issues for the second tutorial.
- What to do when you lose your motivation for learning.
- What to do when you do not understand your textbook.

HOW IS THE BOOK ORGANISED?

The book is divided into four parts:

- *Part One—Introduction to problem-based learning*: sets up the general framework for the book and enlarges your understanding of how problem-based learning is different from traditional learning; the aims of PBL; the essential elements in a PBL course; the keys for successful group discussion and action verbs that can empower group dynamics.
- *Part Two—Study skills in problem-based learning*: introduces you to self-directed learning in PBL courses; shows you how to define your learning issues; illustrates the use of mechanisms and flow charts in PBL; demonstrates how to construct your own mechanism for each case; and supplies the keys for using resources and fostering your learning skills.
- *Part Three—Assessment*: provides you with aims of assessment in a PBL curriculum; the tools commonly used in formative and summative assessment and tips for increasing your scores in examinations.
- *Part Four—The successful student in problem-based learning*: introduces you to non-cognitive skills and professionalism. It also provides you with the keys for success by showing you how to practise the habits of successful people and concentrate on your skills to achieve your dreams.

HOW TO USE THIS BOOK

This is a practical guide to help you develop new learning skills. Throughout you are asked to do a variety of exercises. The aim of these exercises is to change your perspective about learning and allow you to experience new insights that ensure your success. The exercises are designed to help you to realise that:

- there are ways to enhance your learning skills
- by understanding the philosophy of PBL you will be able to shape your learning strategies effectively
- successful learning can be developed by applying the tips discussed in the different chapters of this book.

Some exercises will help you develop your intuitive skills and habits, others provide regular checks to polish these skills and some are designed to help you plan to achieve your goals.

Keep a reflective journal

Creative individuals often keep journals to record their thoughts and observations. In PBL it is important to record your responses to the exercises included in this book. Such a journal is usually called a *reflective journal*. Not only will this allow you to reflect on and analyse your learning strategies, but it will also help you to improve your skills, change your attitude and acquire new learning competencies.

Reflective journals will help you to achieve these goals by:

- identifying your areas of strength and those that need improvement
- planning suitable strategies to develop new learning skills
- using motivation to foster your approach
- developing a vision about your short- and long-term goals
- discovering the value of continuous self-monitoring and critical thinking
- developing a passion for learning and success.

To get an overview of this book, skim the contents or flip through the pages and when you see a topic of interest, stop and read thoroughly. But do not just read what is written; keep asking yourself: 'How can I use the information provided?', 'What strategies should I use?', 'How can the new strategies help me?', 'How can I tell?', 'What might prevent me from using these strategies?' Thinking about these questions as you read will help you get the best from the book. I have included critical questions, boxes of ancillary information, inspiring quotes and tips and resources to help you understand the issues discussed and to learn more about applying these strategies. A number of chapters end with an evidence-based learning box, the aim of which is to provide you with the best available evidence on issues raised in the chapter so you can use research to improve your learning.

This book does not provide a quick fix for your problems or areas of deficiency. To achieve your goals, you need to change your learning style, enhance your learning skills and develop new skills. You need to experiment, try new strategies, monitor your progress, learn from your mistakes and persist in the face of setbacks.

Good luck

Samy Azer

email: azer2000@optusnet.com.au

About the author

PROFESSOR SAMY AZER
MB, BCh, MSc Medicine, MEd (NSW), PhD (Syd), FACG, MPH (NSW)

Samy Azer is the Professor of Medical Education at the Faculty of Medicine, the Universiti Teknologi MARA, Malaysia. He is a Visiting Professor of Medical Education, School of Medicine, the University of Toyama, Japan. From 1999 to 2006 he was a Senior Lecturer in Medical Education, Faculty of Medicine, Dentistry and Health Sciences, the University of Melbourne. Professor Azer has trained more than 500 educators from the University of Melbourne and four other Australian universities. He has helped his trainees introduce problem-based learning (PBL) into a number of courses including medicine, physiotherapy, nursing, speech pathology, occupational therapy, dentistry, nutrition, basic sciences, veterinary sciences, as well as secondary and primary education. Prior to 1999, he was Senior Lecturer in Medical Education at the School of Medicine, the University of Sydney.

Professor Azer has a longstanding research interest in medical education, particularly in the areas of curriculum structure and design, enhancement of the facilitation skills of PBL tutors, PBL group dynamics, the role of the scribe in PBL, innovation in assessment and writing questions and testing students' cognitive skills. He has been keynote speaker and a scholar at a number of universities including Universiti Teknologi MARA, Malaysia; Kaohsiung Medical University, Taiwan and the University of Toyama, Japan.

He is the convener of the Problem-Based Learning Special-Interest Group of the Australian and New Zealand Health Association for Health Education (ANZAME). He is also the author of a textbook on assessment for medical students, *Core Clinical Cases in Basic Biomedical Science: Problem-Based Learning Approach*, (Hodder Arnold, 2006) and two categories—internal medicine and gastroenterology—in *Mosby's Dictionary of Medical, Nursing & Health Professions* (Elsevier, 2006). He has contributed to the online chapters of *Kumar & Clark's Clinical Medicine* (Elsevier, 2005) and four chapters in *eMedicine*, the largest international online medical textbook. He is also the author and creator of a multimedia CD-ROM used as a resource by medical students in a number of universities, *The Liver: Understanding Bile Salts and Bilirubin Metabolism* (University of Melbourne, 2005).

Acknowledgments

The author would like to thank students, PBL tutors and colleagues who provided encouragement, advice, information, criticism and support during the preparation of this book. In particular I thank medical and physiotherapy students at the University of Melbourne for their motivation to write this book. I thank my daughter Diana Azer for her talent in reviewing the whole manuscript and her valuable comments. I thank the following international reviewers for their comments and feedback; each reviewer commented on one chapter and their feedback helped me adjust the book to satisfy the needs of international students as well.

Professor Mansour Al-Nozha
President of Tibah University and Professor of Medicine
Kingdom of Saudi Arabia

Dr Gudrun Edgren
Senior Lecturer in Medical Education
Center for Teaching and Learning
Faculty of Medicine
Lund University, Sweden

Dr Willem de Grave
Department of Educational Development & Research
Maastricht University, the Netherlands

Professor Hossam Hamdy
Vice-Chancellor for Medical Colleges and Dean, College of Medicine
University of Sharjah, United Arab Emirates

Associate Professor Schinichiro Hirokawa
Vice Director, Maternity and Perinatal Care Center
The University of Toyama, Japan

Professor Sadanobu Kagamimori
Dean, School of Medicine
The University of Toyama, Japan

Professor Isao Kitajima
Department of Clinical Laboratory and Molecular Pathology
The University of Toyama, Japan

Professor Keh-Min Liu
Associate Dean, College of Medicine,
Kaohsiung Medical University, Taiwan

Assistant Professor Patricia Sexton
AT Still University of Health Sciences, USA

Dr Grace Pertiwi Sundari
Chief Executive Officer
Siloam Hospitals Lippo, Indonesia

Associate Professor Seiji Yamada
Hawaii/Pacific Basin Area Health Education Center and Office of Medical Education
John A Burns School of Medicine
University of Hawaii, USA

Professor Seiji Yamashiro
Professor of General Medicine
The University of Toyama, Japan

Professor Dato' Dr Khalid Yusoff
Foundation Dean
Faculty of Medicine
Universiti Teknologi MARA, Malaysia

Professor Datin Dr Khatijah Yusoff
Deputy Vice-Chancellor
Universiti Putra Malaysia, Malaysia

Professor Allyn Walsh
Department Education Coordinator
Department of Family Medicine
McMaster University, Canada

Parts of Ch 3 have been adapted and reproduced with permission from the publisher: Azer SA. Becoming a student in a PBL course: twelve tips for successful group discussion. Med Teach 2004; 26(1):12–15. Parts of Ch 6 have been adapted and reproduced with permission from the publisher: Azer SA. Facilitation of students' discussion in problem-based learning tutorials to create mechanisms: the use of five key questions. Ann Acad Med 2005; 34(8):492–498.

I also thank Ms Lou Thorn, Territory Manager Victoria/South Australia, Elsevier Australia for her support of the very early idea for this book and her continuing encouragement in the writing of it; Ms Sophie Kaliniecki, Publishing Editor, Elsevier Australia for her support of the book and her encouragement during the writing process; Ms Sunalie Silva, Developmental Editor for her skills and innovative work in producing a wonderful resource for PBL students; Ms Helena Klijn, Publishing Services Manager; Ms Lauren Allsop, Editorial Coordinator; Ms Sybil Kesteven, Editor, and all those involved in the design and production for their insight and creativity in producing such a well-crafted learning resource.

PART ONE

INTRODUCTION TO PROBLEM-BASED LEARNING

CHAPTER 1

Problem-based learning overview

Minds are like parachutes. They only function when they are open.
SIR JAMES DEWAR

INTRODUCTION

In the last twenty years there have been significant changes in our world including the rapid accumulation of new knowledge, significant technological changes, great scientific discoveries, as well as the rise of new psychosocial and ethical/moral challenges such as organ donation, cloning, euthanasia, stem cell research, DNA banking, and genetic discrimination.

These changes raise a number of questions with regard to teaching and learning strategies in our universities and schools:

- Will traditional teaching suit the needs of current learners?
- Will it equip them with the skills and competencies required in the workplace?
- Will learners be able to cope with rapid changes in knowledge and technology?
- With the accumulation of new knowledge in different disciplines and different aspects of life, who will teach students to become life-long learners?
- Will traditional teaching approaches prepare them for these challenges?

The aim of this chapter is to respond to these questions and to understand the reasons for moving from traditional teaching to problem-based learning (PBL) or case-based learning (CBL), how these new methods differ from traditional teaching and what the educational aims of a PBL curriculum are.

WHY DO WE USE PROBLEM-BASED LEARNING?

Although traditional teaching of medicine has served us well for almost a century, in the last 20–30 years changes in our understanding of the role of science in relation to health and illness have prompted a re-think of medical education strategies.

The traditional approach in medical and other healthcare courses has been criticised for a number of reasons. Major areas of criticism can be summarised as follows:

- Academic institutions in the first two years of traditional medical and other healthcare courses usually focus on scientific research rather than on the competencies and skills needed in the profession. As a result, students may spend too much time acquiring knowledge that is subsequently forgotten or found to be irrelevant in their future career.
- The traditional approach creates divisions between basic sciences, psychosocial, ethical and moral issues and clinical sciences.

- Traditional courses focus on factual knowledge. Students have to learn detailed information about basic sciences without understanding the purpose for learning these details. Therefore, the application of the knowledge acquired from basic sciences to the clinical situation can be difficult as students do not immediately discuss the clinical significance of the information they have learnt.
- Reports from several countries, for example, the Toronto consensus statement (Simpson et al 1991), have indicated that medical professionals do not display the interactional skills necessary for achieving optimal patient outcomes. This has been related to inadequacies in traditional undergraduate medical education.

In addition to these limitations of a traditional curriculum, a number of other factors have confirmed the need for innovation in medical and other healthcare courses. These factors can be summarised as:

- The need to address changes in our communities, for example, adopting patient-centred healthcare that includes enhanced patient access to information about health and to new developments in diagnosis and therapeutic options.
- The information explosion in medicine and related disciplines and developments in information technology with particular relevance to medical, health, pharmacy and biomedical informatics.
- The need for healthcare professionals to be competent not just in the pathophysiological bases of diseases (the process by which these diseases occur), diagnosis or management of diseases but also in non-cognitive skills such as interpersonal and communication skills, empathy, professionalism, teamwork, integrity and commitment.
- The changing organisational structure in the healthcare system and the need for multi-professional education to enhance collaborative work with other professional groups within health.

As a result of these changes, many international authorities have recommended new guidelines for medical education (e.g. the Edinburgh Declaration of the World Federation for Medical Education, 1988; the World Summit on Medical Education, 1994; the ministerial consultation of the World Health Organization and the World Federation for Medical Education, 1989). These authorities argued that changes were needed in medical and related curricula to establish learning environments that match the professional activities expected from learners. To achieve these goals, they supported the introduction of integrated PBL or CBL and a multi-professional approach.

PBL and multi-professional training provide an ideal strategy to close the gap between education and practice. This is because the focus in PBL is on the students' learning instead of the teaching and by facilitation and self-directed learning it enables students to create their own learning approach.

The primary goals of PBL in medical and related courses are to foster clinical reasoning, problem-solving skills, self-directed learning, communication skills and deep understanding of concepts and principles in the curriculum. This approach was first introduced in the School of Medicine at McMaster University in Canada in 1969. A few years later, two universities adapted the PBL approach to medical education, the University of Limburg at Maastricht in the Netherlands in 1974 and the University of Newcastle in Australia in 1976. Since then the use of PBL in medical education has been endorsed by the Word Health Organization, the Association of American Medical Colleges and the World Federation of Medical Education. PBL is currently the main educational approach used in medical schools in Africa and Asia/Pacific nations, Europe, the Middle East, the United States, and most universities in Australia.

The PBL approach is based on cognitive psychology and the broad principles of self-directed learning. This approach differs fundamentally from the traditional approach in which students acquire knowledge of the basic sciences in the early years of their medical course and apply this knowledge to the diagnosis and management of clinical cases in the last two years of their course.

PBL is widely used in medicine, dental science, forensic examination, nursing, occupational therapy, physiotherapy and speech pathology. It is also used in non–health courses such as accounting, architecture, economics, engineering, law and policing. The teacher in a PBL course is a facilitator rather than an information provider. Thus, their role is completely different from that of a traditional teacher. In addition, students assume considerable responsibility for their own learning and they play an active role in the discussion of the PBL case.

TRADITIONAL AND PROBLEM-BASED CURRICULA

Before discussing your roles in PBL, let us have an overall look at the two types of curricula.

The design of the curriculum is vital to the effectiveness of PBL because the design affects the interaction between students and teachers, their responsibilities and their roles during curriculum delivery. Table 1.1 summarises four levels of student/teacher interactions in a curriculum.

Level 1: traditional way of teaching where the teacher is the authority figure and the source of information; the student is dependent on the teacher. A good example of this level of curriculum structure is the traditional curriculum which encourages passive learning and uses lecture-based education.

Level 2: the situation where some improvements have been added to enhance a traditional curriculum, for example, using interactive lectures and introducing some strategies to enhance students' motivation.

Levels 3 and 4: the other side of the spectrum where the teacher is a facilitator, feedback provider and delegator, while the student takes the lead and uses self-directed learning strategies. Good examples for levels 3 and 4 of curriculum structure are PBL, CBL, case-based reasoning, and use of computer-aided learning programs.

TABLE 1.1 The four levels of student/teacher interaction in a curriculum			
Level	**Student**	**Teacher**	**Examples**
Level 1	Dependent	Authority, information provider	Passive learning. Lecture-based teaching encouraging rote learning.
Level 2	Interested	Motivator, guide	Inspiring lecture with occasional guided discussion.
Level 3	Takes the lead	Facilitator, feedback provider	PBL, CBL, case-based reasoning, and other types of small group learning.
Level 4	Self-directed	Delegator, consultant	Self-directed study, e.g. using computer-aided programs.

In PBL, you will be working in a small group of students on a written case *scenario* (problem). For these cases you will need to work with other students in your group to identify the problems, generate *hypotheses* (possible causes), and look for more information (construct an *enquiry plan*) to refine your hypotheses. However, during this process, you will discover that you have *learning issues* (gaps in your knowledge) and need to research these questions and find appropriate answers. You then have to research your own identified learning issues, report back to your group, and apply the knowledge you have learnt to the case. All the work is done by you and other members in the group. Your tutor's role is to facilitate group discussion. (See Ch 3 for more details about your tutor's role.)

THE STUDENT'S ROLE

Now let us look at your role in a problem-based curriculum and how your roles are different from those in a traditional curriculum.

In PBL:

- You learn how to apply knowledge to real–life situations, while in a traditional course you learn how to focus on factual knowledge.
- You become producers of information (construct information), while in a traditional course you consume knowledge.
- You ask questions and research for answers, while in a traditional course your teacher asks, and may answer, all questions.
- You research your own resources, while in a traditional course you rote learn the knowledge given to you.
- You actively analyse information, while in a traditional course you sometimes accept knowledge as it is.
- You actively work in small groups, while in a traditional course you listen passively to lectures with a large number of students.
- You learn from other students, while in a traditional course you learn from your teacher.
- You learn by cooperation, while in a traditional course you learn by competition.
- You learn for understanding, while in a traditional course you learn for examinations.
- You learn to elaborate on what you learnt, while in a traditional course you learn to memorise facts.
- You see the relevance of knowledge learnt, while in a traditional course you sometimes struggle with dry information (for example, you are not clear about its use in your career and its applications).
- You rely on a wide range of learning resources while in a traditional course you use the recommended textbook.

Other aspects of PBL and how it differs from traditional teaching are discussed in 'The aims of PBL' later in this chapter.

DEFINING PROBLEM-BASED LEARNING

In PBL, learning results from the process of working toward the understanding or resolution of a problem. The problem is encountered first in the learning process and serves as a focus or stimulus for the application of problem solving or reasoning skills, as well as for the search for or study of information or knowledge needed to understand the mechanisms responsible for the problem and how it might be resolved. HOWARD BARROWS AND ROBYN TAMBLYN

If anyone has told you what 'PBL' means, chances are the definition was vague or confusing. The fact is nobody agrees on a single definition. Different schools have adopted their own model and define PBL as per their model.

You could argue that the word 'problem' refers to the case used in the tutorials and to the patient's problems as identified by the students. You could also argue that 'problem' refers to the fact that the case is written in a problem format with a lot of uncertainty (ill-structured) and that students need to work together to solve the problem. A third possibility could be that the questions raised during the discussion of the case are the *real* 'problems' that need to be researched by students. As a result we see many different definitions of PBL in the literature. However, I believe that these definitions complement each other and each one reflects a specific aspect of PBL. Here are a few examples.

DEFINITIONS FROM THE LITERATURE

Barrows, 1986: 'The term applies to any method that achieves four important objectives in medical education: the structure of knowledge for use in clinical contexts, the development of an effective clinical reasoning process, the development of self-directed learning skills and increasing motivation for learning.'

Albanese and Mitchell, 1993: 'It is crucial that the problem raise compelling issues for new learning and that students have an opportunity to become actively involved in the discussion of these issues, with appropriate feedback and corrective assistance from faculty members.'

Vernon and Blake, 1993: 'PBL is a method of learning or teaching that emphasizes the study of clinical cases, either real or hypothetical; small group discussion; collaborative independent study; hypothetical–deductive reasoning and a style of learning that concentrates on group process rather than imparting information.'

Schmidt, 1993: 'An approach to learning and instruction in which students tackle problems in small groups under supervision of a tutor.'

From these definitions we can conclude that the existing definitions of PBL have several problems:

- They focus on different aspects in PBL.
- They might complement each other.
- They do not explain what is meant by a problem. Is it the patient's problem? Is it the learning problems? Or is it both?

DEFINITIONS FROM STUDENTS

Recently, I asked a group of medical and physiotherapy students to write down what they understand from the term PBL and how they perceive PBL as a learning method. These students have been using PBL in their learning for over a year. These are some of their responses.

Caitlin, 2nd-year medical student: 'The first case we had was different from anything I have ever learnt. We were not sure. We asked a lot of questions. Everyone in the group was working hard. We tried to explain things and make conclusions. I think this lack of knowledge kept everyone engaged in the process. When I started searching for answers for our questions, I was really very eager to find out information about the problem. The more I researched the more I got more clues and I felt satisfied. This was different from the way I used to learn in high school.'

Sarah, 2nd-year medical student: 'Because we did not know and the tutor did not help us, I was really sceptical about PBL and its value. But after two or three sessions, I started to realise how the discussion in PBL was valuable, particularly when we did not agree on an issue and start sharing ideas. The way we work together as a group is also useful because everyone feels that it is their own learning and we have to be accountable and use the tutorial time effectively.'

Kevin, 2nd-year physiotherapy student: 'Through the discussion of the case I learnt a lot from the contribution of other members in the group. Sometimes I felt I misunderstood what a lecturer said or what I read in textbooks, but through the questions we raised in the tutorial and the input of everyone, we gained a better understanding of the new concepts discussed. I do not think lectures would have provided me with such opportunities.'

THE AIMS OF PROBLEM-BASED LEARNING

> PBL requires students to become responsible for their own learning. The PBL teacher is a facilitator of student learning, and his/her interventions diminish as students progressively take on responsibility for their own learning processes.
>
> CINDY HMELO-SILVER AND HOWARD BARROWS

The main educational objectives of PBL can be summarised as follows: use of problems to acquire a knowledge base that is easy to retain; development of the clinical reasoning and problem-solving skills characteristic of the expert clinician; development of self-directed learning skills; development of a professional attitude and non-cognitive skills such as empathy, communication and interpersonal skills; provision of a student-centred learning approach; and encouragement of independent critical thinking skills.

LEARNING THROUGH PROBLEMS

One of the differences between PBL and traditional teaching is the use of problems (cases) to encourage students' thinking and engagement. Although many courses maintain the effective delivery of lectures, in a PBL curriculum, lectures are not the primary source of teaching and they are usually designed in a new format that encourages thinking and understanding rather than factual knowledge and rote learning. The scenarios are written in an innovative way to keep learners thinking about the situation and people involved in the case scenario. They are also created in a way that suits the learners' age group, culture, prior knowledge and expectations. Course designers ensure that the scenarios are carefully written with no ambiguity and reflect the educational objectives allocated for the case.

Why do we use case scenarios?

- Scenarios allow students to reflect upon what they can do and think about approaches to collect new information to solve a problem.
- Scenarios attempt to situate learning in contexts that are similar to what learners face in their real-life situations. On this basis, a learner when faced with a novel case scenario can use their knowledge to assist understanding of the different dimensions of a problem.
- Scenarios allow students to generate hypotheses for the problems, and think about approaches to make priorities between their hypotheses.

- Scenarios serve as a vehicle for integrating knowledge and linking basic sciences with clinical situations.
- Scenarios allow students to discuss moral and ethical issues raised in the case scenario.
- Scenarios aid the retention of information in the long-term memory.
- Scenarios allow students to provide evidence and reasoning for their views/actions.
- Scenarios stimulate and excite the students and make them want to learn further.

ACHIEVING INTEGRATION

In a traditional course students study each discipline separately. For example, students may commence their first year studying disciplines such as anatomy, physiology, biochemistry, and histology. Each of these subjects is taught on its own. This approach is not encouraged in PBL or case-based curricula. One of the goals of PBL is to achieve integration. This goal is achieved through the use of case scenarios. The use of case scenarios encourages the learner to discuss the problem and search for solutions. To do this students research and study issues from different disciplines such as anatomy, biochemistry, microbiology, pharmacology, physiology and medicine. They might also discuss moral and ethical issues raised in the case. In this way, PBL enhances students' critical thinking, reasoning and weighing of evidence before making decisions. It develops deep understanding across disciplines of the concepts raised in the problem. Table 1.2 shows how learning in an integrated curriculum differs from learning in a traditional curriculum.

ACHIEVING COGNITIVE OBJECTIVES

One of the primary aims of PBL is keeping the learner motivated and interested in researching for more information related to the case, rather than merely solving the problem. Case scenarios are designed to develop a number of cognitive skills including:
- generating hypotheses
- refining hypotheses on the basis of evidence available from history and clinical examination
- enhancing critical thinking
- integrating basic and clinical sciences as well as psychosocial issues and ethical/moral concepts with other issues raised from the case discussion
- using basic sciences to understand clinical signs and patient's presenting symptoms
- providing justification for the changes observed
- providing an interpretation of clinical findings and investigation results
- dealing with uncertainty and learning the art of decision making
- designing a management plan—defining goals for the management plan and the best available options.

What are the advantages of mastering these cognitive skills rather than just focusing on factual knowledge?
- Hmelo (1998) in an excellent study addressed this question. In her study, students in full-time PBL, elective PBL and full-time traditional curricula at two schools were compared on a series of pathophysiological explanation tasks over the course of the first year of medical school. The students' ability to solve

TABLE 1.2 Comparison: learning in an integrated curriculum and in a traditional curriculum	
An integrated curriculum helps students to:	**In a discipline-based curriculum students tend to:**
See the significance and clinical uses of basic sciences	See the clinical use of basic sciences in later years of the course
Use information from several disciplines as they discuss the case and prepare their learning issues	Learn in a frame bounded by each discipline
Integrate information, e.g. build mechanisms, assess the pathogenesis of diseases	Learn issues related to a discipline
Consider moral, psychosocial and ethical issues in their management plan	Focus on the disease and ignore issues related to the patient
Use basic sciences in their reasoning	Be less likely to use basic sciences learnt in the early years of their course

problems was considered from several viewpoints such as accuracy, coherence and comprehensiveness of explanation, reasoning strategies and use of science concepts. The data from this study showed that the PBL students generated explanations that were more accurate, coherent and comprehensive than those of non-PBL students. They were able to transfer the reasoning strategies they were taught and were more likely to use scientific concepts in their explanations. This effect was stronger for the full-time PBL students. The author concluded that by promoting the use of hypothesis-driven reasoning strategies, PBL might accelerate this development as students engage knowledge that will eventually become encapsulated under their hypotheses.

- Enhancement of the cognitive skills of the students targets deep understanding whereas focusing on factual knowledge does not provide students with the opportunity to critically analyse information, test their hypotheses and examine the best approaches to solve a problem and make decisions.

PROMOTING SMALL-GROUP LEARNING

One of the objectives of PBL and CBL is promoting small-group learning. A group consists of 8 to 12 students joined by a tutor. Usually a group functions for a semester—about 12–14 weeks—then students move to join newly established groups. This allows students to work with other students in their cohort and maximise their learning and relationships with other students and new tutors. It might be of interest to you to look at Tuckman's work about the five stages of group development (see Box 1.1). This information can help you to be prepared for the different stages your group will go through, reassure you about the changes you will observe in your group as well as help you to be one of the wise members who keep the group moving and functioning through these stages.

What are the advantages of small-group learning?

The small-group format:

- is invaluable in the development of skills such as negotiation, effective communication and collaborative learning

BOX 1.1 Stages of group development

Stage 1: Orientation

During this stage, relations between members are characterised by dependence. The group members seek safe pattern behaviour and look to their PBL tutor for guidance and direction. Members have a drive for acceptance by other members. Serious topics and feelings are avoided by everyone and members are more interested in becoming oriented to the task and to one another.

Stage 2: Struggle

During this stage, members show competition. Some members may have to mould their feelings and beliefs to suit the group function. Fear of exposure may surface. Although struggle may not surface and become apparent to everyone, it does exist. Some members may remain completely silent and ignore the apparent difficulties while others may attempt to dominate the group and take control. Self-control, wisdom, listening to each other, motivation to work together and guidance from the tutor are very important at this stage.

Stage 3: Overcoming the struggle

This stage is characterised by the development of interpersonal relations and cohesion. The level of trust between members has increased and a sense of group belonging is in place. There is also a sense of relief that the group has managed well with their interpersonal conflict during the struggle stage. Members are more engaged and there is more contribution from each member of the group. Leadership is shared and members are open to sharing their feelings, ideas and giving feedback to one another. They are interested in improving their group function and working together. Members may become worried about the inevitable break-up of the group and some may contact staff about their feelings and their willingness to continue with the same group next semester. Members at this stage will resist any changes.

Stage 4: True interdependence

This stage may not be reached by all groups. Groups may break up at stage 3 or 4 by the end of a semester. If the group members are able to evolve to the end of stage 4, their capacity and the depth of their personal relationships will be expanded to true interdependence. All members have become self-assured; they do not feel that they need group approval any more. Group morale is high. Members are productive and focused on achievements. They enjoy working together as well as with other groups.

Stage 5: Completion of the task

This is the last stage; the group by now has completed its function. This is the stage of termination of task behaviour and disengagement from relationships. Each member is recognised for their role in the group and members are acknowledged for their achievements.

Modified from: Tuckman B. Developmental sequence in small groups. Psychol Bull 1965; 63: 384–399; Tuckman B, Jensen M. Stages of small group development. Group Organisation Studies 1977; 2:419–427.

- helps learners build their own knowledge
- enables students to identify gaps in their knowledge and acquire new knowledge to deepen their understanding of a new concept
- is better than a lecture, particularly for higher order activities such as analysis, evaluation, critical thinking, decision making, synthesis and defining learning needs
- provides students with the opportunity to share their views, test their own ideas, and assess their understanding of a concept against those of others

- enhances students' motivation and engagement in learning as they discuss the problem and deal with uncertainty
- forces members of the group to explore issues at a deeper level. Group discussion activates previously acquired understanding, helping identify any deficits and facilitating new comprehensions
- promotes an adult style of learning, and the development of collaborative learning and a number of transferable skills
- provides opportunity to give and receive feedback
- provides opportunity for learners to learn from each other rather than from 'experts' who sometimes cannot explain content at the level needed by the learner.

What are the key attitudes that can improve group function?

Students' positive attitudes towards the group help a great deal in achieving better group function. These may include:

- being committed to the group process
- accepting each member as they are
- demonstrating responsibility for and willingness to spend time and energy on the group
- willingness to work with all members in the group
- monitoring their interaction with other members
- believing in the group
- willingness to share learning resources with other members
- communicating with other members in the group in a constructive way
- being critical at the right time and in the right way.

PROMOTING SELF-DIRECTED LEARNING

Students in small groups work together to identify the key information provided in the case, generate hypotheses, and develop a reasonable approach to working out the problem. During their discussion they identify gaps in their knowledge and raise a number of questions they need to research. These are usually known as *learning issues*. (See Chs 4 and 5 for more detailed information about self-directed learning and learning issues, respectively.)

Self-directed learning is an adult learning strategy. It is information seeking behaviour in response to identified learning needs. This leads to targeted use by the learner of a variety of learning resources to overcome deficiencies in knowledge, skills or professional development. Effective self-directed learning requires the development of self-assessment skills, critical appraisal skills and effective time management. Self-directed learning encourages students to organise their thinking by comparing ideas, analysing information, asking questions and reaching conclusions.

What factors enhance my self-directed learning?
Intrinsic interest in the content to be mastered
Self-motivation in knowledge acquisition
Curiosity to learn and find answers to questions raised during the case discussion
Engagement in the discussion of the case
Good group dynamics
Well-designed PBL cases
Availability of learning resources
Assessment matches the design of the curriculum

What educational resources may I use in a PBL curriculum?
PBL cases
Lectures
Computer-aided learning programs
Journal articles
Textbooks
eBooks and educational websites
Practical classes
Patient education resources
Medical and healthcare societies' educational resources
Anatomy/pathology specimens

PROMOTING TEAMWORK

The multi-professional aspects of contemporary healthcare require teamwork: PBL allows students to work effectively in small groups and develop a good understanding of teamwork, effective communication, and collaborative learning. Transferable skills such as leadership, teamwork, organisational ability, providing support, prioritising and setting goals, problem solving, motivating others and managing time are important attributes in healthcare professionals.

Working in groups provides mutual support and lays the foundations for future behaviour as a professional. Such competencies are best fostered through role modelling (see also Ch 12). Students can observe the effect they have on other members in the group. In PBL programs, which emphasise the importance of early contact with patients and clinicians, students practise communication skills from the first week of their first year and are able to see the importance of role models in clinical education and the significance of teamwork.

What actions foster successful teamwork?
Building trust with other members
Showing acceptance and interest in other people's views
Listening to others
Respecting people with views different from yours
Enhancing group dynamics
Investing in working effectively with other members
Communicating effectively with others
Encouraging people to work with you
Focusing on shared goals in the group
Encouraging feedback on the group's function
Defining the purpose and goals of the group
Sharing your vision with other members
Willingness to discuss problems in the group and find solutions

Why promote teamwork?
Students realise that:
Better outcomes are achieved through teamwork
Healthcare services are based on teamwork
Success in medical and healthcare careers is the result of effective teamwork

CONCLUSIONS

PBL is a student-centred approach that enhances deep learning. The approach uses problems to develop a number of skills including integration of knowledge, cognitive skills, small-group and self-directed learning, teamwork and critical thinking. Compared to those in a traditional curriculum, students in a PBL course play a significant role and have, in large measure, responsibility for the success of their course. The secrets for success in a PBL course and how to turn these principles into action are discussed in Chs 2 to 13.

FURTHER READING
BOOKS

Jaques D. Small group teaching. Oxford Brookes University, Oxford Centre for Staff and Learning Development, 2004. Online. Available: http://www.brookes.ac.uk/services/ocsd/2_learntch/small-group/sgtindex.html; 21 Mar 2007.

David T, Patel L, Burdett K, Rangachari P. Problem-based learning in medicine. A practical guide for students and teachers. Worcester: Royal Society of Medicine Press Ltd; 1999.

ARTICLES AND RESEARCH PAPERS

Albanese MA, Mitchell S. Problem-based learning: a review of literature on its outcomes and implementation issues. Acad Med 1993; 68(1): 52–81.

Barrows HS. A taxonomy of problem-based learning methods. Med Educ 1986; 20(6): 481–486.

Bligh JG. Problem based, small group learning. BMJ 1995; 311(7001): 342-343.

Custers EJF, Cate OT. Medical students' attitudes towards and perception of the basic sciences: a comparison between students in the old and the new curriculum at the University Medical Center Utrecht, The Netherlands. Med Educ 2002; 36(12):1142–1150.

Dolmans DH, Schmidt HG. What drives the student in problem-based learning? Med Educ 1994; 28(5):372–380.

Hmelo CE. Cognitive consequences of problem-based learning for the early development of medical expertise. Teach Learn Med 1998; 10:92–100.

Hmelo-Silver CE. Problem-based learning: what and how do students learn? Educ Psych Review 2004; 16:235–266.

Jaques D. Teaching small groups. BMJ 2003; 326(7387):492–494.

Jowett N, LeBlanc V, Xeroulis G, et al. Surgical skill acquisition with self-directed practice using computer-based video training. Am J Surg 2007; 193:237–242.

Kaufman DM, Holmes DB. Tutoring in problem-based learning: perceptions of teachers and students. Med Educ 1996; 30(5):371–377.

Leggat SG. Effective healthcare teams require effective team members: defining teamwork competencies. BMC Health Serv Res 2007; 7:7-17.

Loyens S, Rikers R, Schmidt H. Students' concepts of constructivist learning: a comparison between a traditional and a problem-based learning curriculum. Adv Health Sci Educ Theory Prac 2006; 11(4):365–379.

Maudsley G. Making sense of trying not to teach: an interview study of tutors' ideas of problem-based learning. Acad Med 2002; 77(2):162–172.

McLean M, Van Wyk JM, Peters-Futre EM, et al. The small group in problem-based learning: more than a cognitive 'learning' experience for first-year medical students in a diverse population. Med Teach 2006; 28(4):e94–e103(1).

Peile ED. Integrated learning. BMJ 2006; 332(7536):276.

Schmidt HG. Foundations of problem-based learning: some explanatory notes. Med Educ 1993; 27(5):422–432.

Simpson M, Buckman R, Stewart M, et al. Doctor–patient communication: the Toronto consensus statement. BMJ 1991; 303(6814):1385–1387.

Tuckman B. Developmental sequence in small groups. Psychol Bull 1965; 63:384–399.

Tuckman B. Jensen M. Stages of small group development. Group Organisation Studies 1977; 2:419–427.

Van Berkel HJM, Schmidt HG. Motivation to commit oneself as a determinant of achievement in problem-based learning. Higher Educ 2000; 40(2):231–242.

Vernon DT, Blake RL. Does problem-based learning work? A meta-analysis of evaluative research. Acad Med 1993; 68(7):550–563.

Williamson SN. Development of a self-rating scale of self-directed learning. Nurse Res 2007; 14(2):66–83.

Wood DF. ABC of learning and teaching in medicine: Problem based learning. BMJ 2003; 326(7384): 328–330.

World Federation for Medical Education. Proceedings of the World Summit on Medical Education. Med Educ 1994; 28:S1.

World Federation for Medical Education. The Edinburgh Declaration. Lancet 1988; 8068:464.

World Health Organization/World Federation for Medical Education. Ministerial Consultation on Medical Education EUR/ICP/HMD/115. Copenhagen: WHO Regional Office for Europe; 1989.

CHAPTER 2

Problem-based learning cases

> The important thing is not to stop questioning. Curiosity has its own reason for existing. **ALBERT EINSTEIN**

INTRODUCTION

Problem-based learning (PBL) cases are usually discussed in two or three tutorials; each of which is two hours long. However, this is not a strict rule and schools may structure their PBL cases differently depending on their students' needs, the design of the curriculum, and their teaching strategies. Each case starts with a 'trigger', a text of 5–6 lines that may be accompanied by an image, a series of images, a short video clip, or even a cartoon.

The educational objectives in tutorial 1 are to:

1 Identify key information in the trigger text and image(s).
2 Identify the patient's problem(s) from the information provided in the trigger.
3 Generate a list of hypotheses for each problem identified.
4 Develop an *enquiry plan* that could provide further information from the history. The aim is to ask the patient or their relatives questions that could make the hypotheses less likely, more likely or cause them to be excluded. As the case progresses, the group may seek further information via clinical examinations or laboratory investigations to refine the final hypothesis.
5 Use information from basic sciences (e.g. biology, psychology or sociology) to build mechanisms that explain each hypothesis.
6 Formulate the learning issues of the case. During the discussion of the case, members of the group may discover they have gaps in their knowledge in relation to the concepts and principles discussed. The group may agree on 5–6 key learning issues and phrase these issues in question form. At the end of tutorial 1, each student in the group will take these learning issues away to research appropriate new knowledge to bring to the group in tutorial 2.

The educational objectives of tutorial 2 are to:

1 Discuss learning issues identified in tutorial 1 and use the knowledge gained from textbooks and computer-aided programs since tutorial 1 to explain issues raised in the case.
2 Identify laboratory tests and other investigations that could help refine the hypotheses.
3 Analyse, evaluate and interpret the data provided in investigation results.
4 Refine the hypotheses and identify evidence from the history, clinical examination and investigations that supports these views.

5 Discuss overall management goals, available options and factors that may interfere with each option.

6 In the last 10 minutes, group members may discuss how they have worked as a team and provide suggestions to improve performance in next week's tutorial.

As mentioned, schools may structure their PBL cases differently and address these educational objectives using different strategies. There are several types of problems used in medicine and other healthcare courses. Therefore, the structure of the PBL cases used in your institution may not match the case outlined in this chapter. However, the basic principles are usually the same.

TUTORIAL 1: ESSENTIAL ELEMENTS

In this section, I address in detail the essential elements of PBL cases for this tutorial. Figure 2.1 summarises the steps in tutorial 1.

1. TRIGGER

A trigger initiates a problem. It is usually a brief text that includes 3–4 keywords. It may be accompanied by an image, a series of images, a video clip, or even a cartoon. The group brainstorms to identify key information and the patient's problems.

Example of a trigger

You are a medical student undertaking a clinical rotation with Dr Albert Waterman in the outpatient clinic. Mrs Lillian Thomson, a 65-year-old retired primary school teacher, comes in with her daughter to see Dr Waterman. Mrs Thomson has had three episodes of upper abdominal pain over the last 24 hours. On her way to the clinic, she vomited twice. She says, 'My urine has become dark over the last few hours'.

Discussion questions
• List the key information about Mrs Thomson.
• List Mrs Thomson's presenting problem(s).
Summarise your answers to these questions.

Answers
Key information

A 65-year-old retired primary school teacher

Presented to her GP with 3 attacks of abdominal pain over the last 24 hours.

She vomited twice

Her urine is dark in colour

Problems

Abdominal pain: 3 attacks

Vomited twice

Dark urine

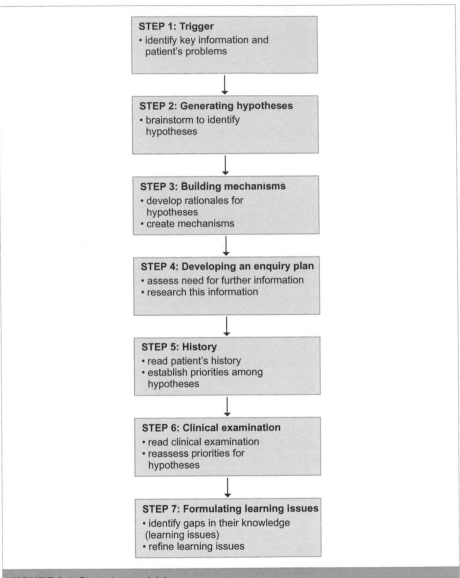

FIGURE 2.1 Steps in tutorial 1.

What are the educational aims of the trigger?
- Stimulate students to identify patient's problems.
- Provide key information about patient's background.
- Allow students to meet the patient in the case.
- Foster students' observation skills by use of images that accompany the trigger text.

2 GENERATING HYPOTHESES

At this stage, the group identifies the hypotheses for each problem. This is a brainstorming process; every student in the group should contribute. The *scribe*, one of the students in the group, organises this information on the board. The tutor might ask key questions to foster discussion at this stage.

Discussion question
• What are the hypotheses for each problem identified?
Summarise your answer to this question.
    If students are unable to answer this question, that is, are unable to state a reasonable number of hypotheses (about 6 or 7 causes), the tutor might ask students more questions to facilitate the discussion of the original question. Look at these questions:
1 What are the structures in the upper abdomen and the lower part of the chest that could be the source of Mrs Thomson's pain?
2 What could possibly go wrong with each of these structures to produce pain?
3 List hypotheses for each of Mrs Thomson's problems.

Answers
Hypotheses for each of her problems:

Abdominal pain
    Stomach ulcer
    Duodenal ulcer
    Gastritis (inflammation of the stomach)
    Heart attack
    Gallbladder problems (for example, a stone moving into the bile duct)

Vomiting
    Inflammation of the stomach
    Gastroenteritis (infection)
    Ear problem (causing reflex contraction of the stomach and vomiting)
    Intestinal obstruction

Dark urine
    Blood in urine
    Concentrated urine (dehydrated)
    Metabolites excreted in urine
  1 Structures that might be the source of her pain
    Stomach
    Duodenum
    Heart
    Lung
    Pleura
    Pancreas
    Liver
    Gallbladder
    Colon

Abdominal wall, including ribs

2 What could possibly go wrong with each structure producing pain?

Stomach ⇨ inflammation of its lining, ulcer

Duodenum ⇨ ulcer

Heart ⇨ lack of oxygen supply to its muscle (heart attack)

Pleura ⇨ inflammation

Pancreas ⇨ inflammation (e.g. pancreatitis)

Liver ⇨ inflammation, pressure on its capsule

Gallbladder ⇨ inflammation of its wall, gallstones in the bile duct

Colon ⇨ inflammation of the colon, constipation

Muscle wall, including ribs ⇨ skeletal muscle strain, tear and rib fracture

---

What are the educational objectives of hypotheses generation?
- Thinking about possible causes for the patient's problems.
- Identifying areas that students do not know and about which they might need to find more information.
- Integrating knowledge from basic sciences such as anatomy and physiology with pathology and clinical presentation.
- Using these hypotheses as the basis for the enquiry plan and collection of information from history.
- Training students to use this scientific approach when they face similar problems.

---

3 BUILDING MECHANISMS

The group will be asked at this stage to use their knowledge to develop a rationale or mechanism to explain each of their hypotheses. *Mechanisms* are often a sequence of events linked by arrows. The group might consider in their mechanisms contributing factors including psychosocial issues, body systems and cellular and molecular bases. The group may discover during this process that they lack information in areas such as anatomy, biochemistry, microbiology, pathogenesis, pharmacology or physiology to provide an adequate explanation. The group may suggest that these deficiencies in knowledge be included as part of their learning issues list. Some groups might prefer to build their mechanisms *after* discussing their enquiry plan, the medical history and the clinical examination findings.

Discussion question
- Select one of your hypotheses and provide a mechanism for it to explain the cause of Mrs Thomson's problem(s).

Summarise your answer to this question.

Answers
Examples of simple mechanisms (see Chapter 6 for more detail).

1 Eating food contaminated with bacteria ⇨ bacteria and toxins reach the gastrointestinal tract ⇨ inflammation of the stomach ⇨ irritation of the nerves in the stomach lining ⇨ abdominal pain

2 Blockage of the blood supply of the heart ⇨ not enough oxygen to the heart muscle ⇨ may affect cardiac muscle contraction + cardiac muscle not functioning in a normal way + accumulation of waste products in the muscle ⇨ pain

As you build your mechanism, a number of questions might be triggered which need answers. For example, the second mechanism might raise the following questions:

Which artery is blocked?

How is the artery blocked?

What exactly causes it to be blocked?

What are the effects of decreased oxygen supply to the heart muscle?

Why does the heart muscle need oxygen?

Are there any other steps that need to be added?

If you are unable to write a mechanism or you are not sure of your answers read Ch 6.

4 DEVELOPING AN ENQUIRY PLAN

The need for further information

At this stage the group will discover that they need further information from the patients, their relatives or treating doctor to evaluate each of their hypotheses. This new information will be obtained from the history, clinical examination and results of investigations. This information will be disclosed to the group as the case progresses over the two tutorials. But before this information is disclosed to the group, they will be asked to develop an enquiry plan—for example, history questions—and to explain how the information will help them in evaluating each of their hypotheses and making priorities.

Discussion question

• What further information from history questions do you require to help you refine your hypotheses? Explain your reasoning.

Summarise your answer to this question.

Answers

Remember that the aim of this task is to ask questions that will help you to assess your hypotheses and make priorities.

Examples of useful questions:

Have you noticed any relationship between the appearance of pain and eating?

What are the types of food that start the pain?

Does the pain increase with movement or turning to one side?

Does the pain increase when you press with your fingers on your chest or abdomen?

Show me the exact site of the pain.

How long have you had the pain?

How would you describe your pain?

What makes the pain better/worse?

Does the pain go anywhere else?

What else is associated with your pain?

How would you rank your pain out of 10, 10 being the worst pain?

Do you have any past history of similar pain?

Have you had any investigations or treatment before?

How about your family? Any family history of health problems?

5 HISTORY

At this stage the tutor will ask the group to turn to the relevant material and read the history. Read the history below and discuss the significance of the new information for establishing priorities among your hypotheses.

Present illness

Mrs Thomson has had similar abdominal pain approximately three times over the last few days. Today she started to feel the pain about an hour after attending her grandson's birthday party. She describes the pain as severe and constant in nature, mainly in the upper right part of her tummy beneath her ribs and occasionally radiating through to her back. She gives a history of vomiting twice and she has nausea during the time of the pain. She has lost no body weight; her appetite is good except when she is in pain. She gives no history of changes in her bowel motions.

Past medical history
* No history of blood transfusion or recent travel overseas.
* She has no history of urinary stones or urinary tract infection.

Family history
* Her father died of liver cancer at 55 years of age.
* Her mother died at the age of 70 of stroke.
* Her only sister, now 57, is alive and well.
* No family history of blood disease or anaemia.

Tobacco and alcohol

Mrs Thomson has not smoked for ten years. She drinks two glasses of wine on weekends.

Medication

She takes paracetamol (acetaminophen) tablets occasionally for headaches.

Allergies
Nil

Social

Mrs Thomson has been a widow for the last two years. She lives with her married daughter. She used to work as a primary school teacher in a private school.

Discussion questions
* Are there terms you do not know/understand?
* Summarise the key information in the history.
* List any new problems. Rank your hypotheses on the basis of the new information provided in the history.
* For each problem, make a list of hypotheses.
* What further information would you like to elicit from a clinical examination?

Summarise your answers to these questions.

Record the learning issues that you have identified so far.

Answers

New term

Paracetamol (acetaminophen): used to treat mild to moderate pain and fever, including simple headaches and muscle aches.

Problems

> Abdominal pain: 3 times over last few days
> Today she has abdominal pain after attending her grandson's birthday party
> Vomited twice + nausea
> Dark urine

Hypotheses

You might need to think about these questions as you rank your hypotheses:

> What is the significance of the occurrence of her symptoms after attending her grandson's birthday party?
> Could her pain and vomiting be caused by food poisoning?
> But how would you explain her dark urine? How would you explain her episodes of abdominal pain prior to the party?
> What type of food could have precipitated her abdominal pain? Explain your answer.
> What do we need to digest this type of food?
> How could this explain her symptoms?
> Why did the doctor ask her about blood transfusion and travel overseas?
> Why did the doctor ask her about anaemia and blood diseases?

You may rank your hypotheses using +++ for most likely, + for less likely, − for hypotheses that could be excluded and query (?) when you are not sure.

The group may need to discuss each hypothesis and reach a consensus. A scribe will help in facilitating this discussion and the decision-making process.

Further information from clinical examination

> Vital signs e.g. temperature, blood pressure, pulse rate and respiratory rate
> Any signs of chronic liver problems
> Abdominal examination
> Examination of the abdominal wall
> Examination of cardiovascular and respiratory systems

6 CLINICAL EXAMINATION

At this stage the tutor will ask the group to turn to the relevant material and read the clinical examination. Read the clinical examination below and think about the significance of the new findings in making priorities from your hypotheses.

General appearance

Mrs Thomson is in pain. She is obviously jaundiced. She has no skin bruising. She has no signs of malnutrition and has no spider angiomas or palmar erythema. Her height is 165 cm, her weight is 79 kg and her body mass index (BMI) is 29 kg/m^2.

TABLE 2.1 Mrs Thomson's vital signs

Vital sign	Mrs Thomson	Normal range
Blood pressure	140/90	100/60–130/80 mmHg
Pulse rate	90	60–100/min
Respiratory rate	18	12–16/min
Temperature	37	36.6–37.2°C

Abdominal examination
- Tenderness in the right upper abdomen. No guarding
- Spleen is not palpable
- Rectal examination: a clay-coloured stool on the examining gloved finger

Cardiovascular and respiratory systems
Normal

Musculoskeletal system
No tenderness in the spine

Neurological system
Not examined

Discussion questions
- Are there terms you do not know/understand?
- Summarise the key information in the history.
- List any new problems that can be added to the original problems you have already identified.
- For each problem, make a list of hypotheses.
- What is your most likely hypothesis? Explain your reasons.
- List your learning issues.

Summarise your answers to these questions.
Record and amend your learning issues.

Answers
New terms

Malnutrition: faulty nutrition due to inadequate intake or a metabolic abnormality.

Spider angiomas and palmar erythema: conditions of the skin that are signs of chronic liver disorder.

Body mass index (BMI): body weight (kg)/(height in metres)^2. According to the classification used in Australia and New Zealand, the acceptable range of BMI is 20–25 kg/m^2; underweight < 20 kg/m^2; overweight >25–30 kg/m^2; obese > 30kg/m^2.

Guarding: spasm of the muscle occurring as the body's protection against further injury. Abdominal guarding is a sign of acute peritonitis.

Jaundice: yellow pigmentation of the skin and eyes due to high blood levels of bilirubin.

See Ch 7 for how to use medical dictionaries effectively.

Key information

   Patient is jaundiced
   No signs of malnutrition or chronic liver disease (no palmar erythema, no
      spider angiomas, no skin bruising)
   Not feverish
   Tenderness in the right upper abdomen
   No palpable spleen
   No tenderness of abdominal wall/ribs

Problems

   Jaundice
   Tenderness in the right upper abdomen

Hypotheses

A Most likely causes:
   Gallbladder problems (e.g. gallstones, obstruction of bile duct)
B Less likely causes:
   Liver problems
   Colonic problems
   Stomach ulcer
   Duodenal ulcer
   Abdominal/chest wall
   Heart problems
   Lung/pleura problems
   Kidney problems
   Learning issues: see item 7, following.

7 FORMULATING LEARNING ISSUES

During the tutorial process, the group will realise that there are gaps in their knowledge in relation to issues discussed in the case. Members of the group are required to negotiate these issues and define their final learning issues. For example, students need to identify the specific knowledge they should acquire to complete their mechanisms to fully explain the scientific basis and the pathogenesis of the patient's problems and to provide an interpretation of the clinical findings and the results of investigations.

   Refining the learning issues is the final task in tutorial 1 of each case. Consider the following situation.

   The group has identified the learning issues listed below for the case you have just finished reading in tutorial 1. In the last 10 minutes of this tutorial the group is preparing to edit these learning issues. They need to rank the issues so as to keep those that are related to the case which can promote learning and stimulate discussion in the next tutorial and they need help in identifying the learning issues that could be excluded.

   How do you help the group complete these tasks?

Discussion question

Rank and edit the learning issues listed below. Some of these issues may not be suitable for the final hypothesis and need to be omitted. (Time allowed: 8 minutes.)

1 The anatomy of the gastrointestinal system
2 Mechanisms by which pain arises from upper gastrointestinal tract (GIT) structures
3 The pathogenesis of jaundice
4 Mechanisms by which vomiting might occur
5 Structure and function of the upper gastrointestinal tract (GIT)
6 Structure and function of the biliary system
7 What are the symptoms of peptic ulcer?
8 Ischaemic heart disease
9 Causes of dark urine
10 Pharmacology of paracetamol
11 Understanding difficult terms such as spider angiomas or palmar erythema.
Explain your ranking and the reasons underlying your decisions.
What are the characteristics of good learning issues?

Answers
The edited learning issues for this case are:
>   Mechanisms by which pain arises from upper gastrointestinal tract structures
>   The pathogenesis of jaundice
>   Mechanisms by which vomiting might occur
>   Structure and function of the biliary system
>   Causes of dark urine
>   Understanding difficult terms such as spider angiomas or palmar erythema

General comments
Good learning issues should be:
1 Specific and cover the main principles discussed in tutorial 1
2 Integrated across disciplines
3 Preferably formatted as a question
4 Balanced between the big picture and the fine details
5 No more than about five or six items/questions

TUTORIAL 2: ESSENTIAL ELEMENTS
8 DISCUSSION
Learning and psychosocial issues
In tutorial 2, students usually start with a discussion of their learning issues. They will need a scribe and all students in the group should contribute to the discussion. They may discuss different learning issues then link them back to the findings in the case. This will allow them to understand the significance of the information they have identified from the trigger, history and clinical examination. They may spend up to 60 minutes on this part. Figure 2.2 summarises the steps in tutorial 2.

9 INVESTIGATIONS
Interpretation of laboratory test results and their significance
The tutor might ask what investigations the group would like to order for Mrs Thomson at this stage. They explain how each investigation will help. The tutor then asks the students to turn to the results of the investigations Dr Waterman has arranged for

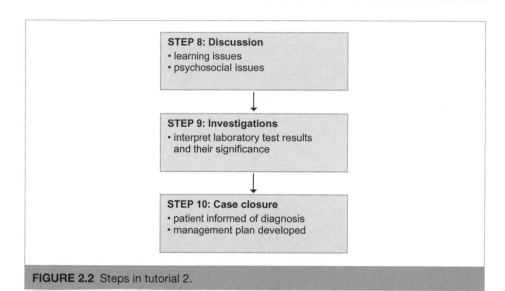

STEP 8: Discussion
• learning issues
• psychosocial issues

STEP 9: Investigations
• interpret laboratory test results
and their significance

STEP 10: Case closure
• patient informed of diagnosis
• management plan developed

FIGURE 2.2 Steps in tutorial 2.

TABLE 2.2 Full blood count results

Blood test	Mrs Thomson	Normal range
Haemoglobin (Hb)	140	115–160 g/L
White blood cell count (WBC)	6.5	$4.0–11.0 \times 10^9$/L
Platelet count	280	$150–400 \times 10^9$/L
Prothrombin time	11	10.5–14.0 s

TABLE 2.3 Liver function tests

Blood test	Mrs Thomson	Normal range
Serum bilirubin	70	0–19 µmol/L
Serum albumin	45	35–50 g/L
Serum alkaline phosphatase (ALP)	340	0–120 U/L
Serum gamma-glutamyl transferase (GGT)	510	0–50 U/L
Serum aspartate aminotransferase (AST)	145	0–40 U/L
Serum alanine aminotransferase (ALT)	130	0–55 U/L

Mrs Thomson to undergo: blood tests and an ultrasound examination of the upper abdomen. The results of these investigations are summarised in Tables 2.2 and 2.3.

Abdominal ultrasound

Common bile duct is 12 mm (normally 3–7 mm). The liver is normal in size and texture. Gallbladder is distended and contains several sonolucent structures identified in the gallbladder with post-sonic shadowing. No stones seen in the cystic duct. The head of the pancreas appears normal but the body and the tail are obscured due to intestinal gases. Kidneys and the aorta are normal.

Discussion questions
- Are there terms you do not know?
- List the abnormalities in these results and any possible causes.
- How does the new information from these investigations help you in refining your hypotheses? Explain your answer.
- Use the information you learnt from basic sciences to construct a mechanism explaining Mrs Thomson's presentation, medical history, findings of the clinical examination and the results of the investigations.

Summarise your answers to these questions.

Answers

New terms
This might vary depending on the number of cases you have studied before studying this case.

The tests may be new to you and you may need to use your textbooks and a medical dictionary to find out more about them (see Chs 7 and 8).

Interpretation of results
The laboratory tests show increased serum bilirubin level (an orange–red pigment formed from haemoglobin during destruction of red blood cells) which explains Mrs Thomson's jaundice (yellow discolouration of her eyes). The increase in serum alkaline phosphatase and gamma-glutamyl transferase is consistent with the presence of cholestasis (stagnation of bile in the liver). This is most likely due to an obstruction of the bile duct. The dilatation of the common bile duct as demonstrated from the abdominal ultrasound confirms the presence of obstruction. Common bile duct obstruction may be caused by: (1) gallbladder stones, (2) enlarged lymph nodes or (3) cancer of the head of the pancreas. The presence of several sonolucent structures identified in the gallbladder with post-sonic shadowing suggests the presence of gallstones. There is no evidence of liver or pancreatic problems. Thus, the final hypothesis is biliary colic caused by gallbladder stones. However, further investigations may be recommended to confirm this.

This case may open the discussion to digestion of fats, the function of the gallbladder, the role of bile salts and pancreatic secretion in digestion of fat, interpretation of liver function tests and the different causes of liver cholestasis.

I would encourage you to read the resources related to this case and build your own mechanism to explain Mrs Thomson's clinical findings and investigation results (see Ch 6).

10 CASE CLOSURE

Dr Waterman explains to Mrs Thomson that the ultrasound scan shows dilatation of the common bile duct. The dilatation usually occurs when there is obstruction of the bile duct. The results of the liver function tests are consistent with this diagnosis. There is no evidence of liver or pancreatic problems. Dr Waterman explains that the obstruction of the bile duct is most likely caused by a stone in the common bile duct. However, this needs confirmation. He adds that the ultrasound examination did not help in identifying the exact cause. An examination using endoscopy called endoscopic retrograde cholangiopancreatography (ERCP) is now needed. The use of ERCP could also help in removing the stone from the common bile duct, if present.

You might search your medical dictionary for these difficult words:

Endoscopic retrograde cholangiopancreatography (ERCP): use of endoscope to visualise the bile duct, biliary system distribution in the liver and the pancreatic duct. The patient is lightly sedated before the procedure and will have little recollection of the event. For more details see: http://www.gastro.org/wmspage.cfm?parm1=860#Expect   See also Figure 2.3.

Papillotomy: incision of the major duodenal papilla. Look at the image of the gallbladder, liver and duodenum at: http://www.healthline.com/adamimage?contentId=1-000273&id=19261&tab=image&series=5&images=7&slide=0

Biliary duct: a tube or channel formed by the union of the common hepatic duct and cystic duct. It conveys the bile from the gallbladder to the duodenum (see also Fig 2.3).

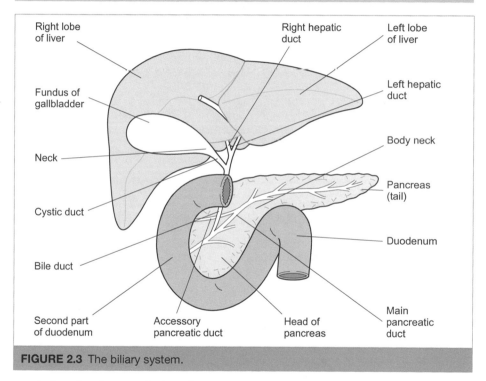

FIGURE 2.3 The biliary system.

A few days later and after obtaining consent from Mrs Thomson, an ERCP is performed and both the pancreatic duct and biliary duct are successfully visualised. Stones are found in the common bile duct, a papillotomy is performed and the stones are removed. Mrs Thomson is observed for 4 hours in the day care department then discharged.

FACILITATING QUESTIONS

Group facilitation is the art of guiding the group process towards the agreed objectives. A facilitator guides the process and does not get involved in content. A facilitator intervenes to protect the group process and keep the group on track to fulfil its task.   DALE HUNTER, ANNE BAILEY AND BILL TAYLOR

The word 'facilitation' has its roots in the French 'faciliter', based on the Latin 'facilis' meaning 'easy'. *Facilitation* is the process of making things easier by making them more efficient or more convenient. In the case of PBL it means helping the group work together and move forward. This includes understanding how the group identifies problems, generates hypotheses, builds mechanisms, debates issues, looks for supportive evidence, solves problems, deals with uncertainty and makes decisions. It also includes how the group handles conflict, assesses their needs and develops strategies to overcome difficulties.

Facilitation is not about detailed content, answering questions or providing a lecture: it is about helping the group deal with big concepts, identifying open-ended questions to encourage group discussion and understanding the learning needs of the group. The facilitator keeps the group focused on their tasks and guides them to achieve their goals.

Your tutor is trained in PBL and in facilitation of group discussion. They will help the group to:
- achieve full cooperation in the discussion and enhance their personal responsibilities in acquiring knowledge and learning
- think critically, communicate clearly and make decisions on the basis of evidence
- develop a number of skills such as interpretation of clinical findings and investigation results, generating hypotheses, building mechanisms, asking good open-ended questions to enhance group discussion and making priorities
- achieve its goals. The tutor will create synergy and promote group cooperation by encouraging each member of the group to contribute, rather than having one person speaking on behalf of all members.

Good open-ended questions used in facilitating group discussion have the following characteristics:
- They stimulate the thinking process.
- They have a purpose and an educational goal.
- They enhance group discussion and help members to deepen their understanding of the concept/issue discussed.
- They allow the group to find new options and expand their discussion.
- They help the group progress and move forward.
- They allow the group to think about resources they might use to get more information.
- They target cognitive skills such as justification, reasoning, lateral thinking and interpretation of findings.

Table 2.4 summarises different types of facilitation questions, their educational aims and provides examples of each type (based on the case of Mrs Thomson).

CONSTRUCTING FACILITATING QUESTIONS

When asking a question, give it some thought so that you phrase it in the best possible way. To do this you might ask yourself these questions:
- Will my question help the current discussion?
- How will my question help the group?
- How might my question enhance our thinking process?
- What does my question target? For example, reasoning knowledge, interpretation knowledge or using lateral thinking.

TABLE 2.4 Questions to facilitate PBL discussion: types, examples and aims

Type of question	Examples	Aims
Finding contributing factors	What are the factors that could have contributed to the appearance of Mrs Thomson's pain after attending the birthday party? How could these factors trigger her pain?	Assess the possible external and internal changes that could be playing a role. Help in deciding which body system is involved. Help in the development of the mechanism. Help in understanding the disease process. Help in making links between the disease process and factors that could be avoided, if possible, when designing the management plan.
Reasoning knowledge	How could food be a contributing factor? What type of food could have precipitated her abdominal pain? Explain your answer. What do we need to digest this type of food? How could this explain her symptoms? Why did the doctor ask her about blood transfusion and travel overseas? Why did the doctor ask her about anaemia and blood diseases?	Provide justification. Provide evidence. Make evidence-based decisions. Explain the underlying scientific basis.
Using lateral thinking	Could her pain and vomiting be caused by food poisoning? But how would you explain her dark urine and jaundice? How would you explain her episodes of abdominal pain prior to the party?	Evaluate hypotheses. Use lateral thinking. Make a decision that considers other findings/information as well.
Source of knowledge	How could we find more information about her presentation? Who could be the source of information?	Deal with uncertainty. Think about resources: relatives (if the patient is unconscious), patient's general practitioner and/or an interpreter (if the patient cannot speak English).
Factual knowledge	What do we know about the liver?	Such questions address rote learning. They might be difficult to be addressed in tutorial 1.

continued

TABLE 2.4 Questions to facilitate PBL discussion: types, examples and aims *continued*

Type of question	Examples	Aims
Procedural knowledge	How can endoscopes be used to remove a biliary stone? Let us describe what can be done.	Describe sequence of events. Describe what the endoscope will do.
	How can endoscopes visualise stones?	Describe the scientific basis of the endoscope.
Interpretation knowledge	What is the significance of her yellow eyes (jaundice)?	Find the changes and think about their significance.
	How can we interpret her pain in light of her jaundice and dark urine?	Choose the best interpretation that could also explain other findings from history, clinical examination and investigation results.
	How can we interpret her ultrasound findings?	
Task-based knowledge	Do we need to find the meaning of these terms?	Use a medical dictionary to find the meaning of difficult words.
	Do we need to search the atlas to find more information about these structures?	Use an atlas to identify specific structures.
	Let us rank our hypotheses using:	Use knowledge created by the group to rank the hypotheses.
	+++ for most likely	
	+ for less likely	
	– for hypotheses that could be excluded	
	query (?) when we are not sure	

- How can I sharpen my question to make it more effective?
- What changes should I consider?

This exercise will help you enhance your ability to ask useful questions that engage your group and foster their thinking. Questions that are well thought out help group discussion, particularly when the group is dealing with a difficult concept or new idea and looking for guidance.

Practise using these questions outside your PBL tutorials so that you become speedy in processing and implementing the steps.

CONCLUSIONS

Not all PBL cases are designed in this format. In some programs, the PBL cases are ill-structured, incompletely specified and may not include a closure. The case discussed in this section is an example of a PBL case presented to students in a progressive way and designed to enhance students' cognitive skills such as: (1) generating hypotheses, (2) building mechanisms, (3) collecting more information from history and clinical examination, (4) selecting priorities from among hypotheses, (5) identifying learning issues, (6) interpreting investigation results, and (7) outlining management goals and options. Some cases may also raise psychosocial concepts and ethical or moral issues. Facilitation questions are useful for group discussion particularly when facing difficult concepts or working on new ideas and looking for guidance. Practising the construction of good open-ended questions will enhance your skills and contribution to the group discussion. It will also foster your self-directed learning skills.

FURTHER READING
BOOKS

Barrows HS. Problem-based learning applied to medical education. Rev edn. Springfield, Ill: Southern Illinois University School of Medicine; 2000.

Barrows HS, Tamblyn RM. Problem-based learning: an approach to medical education. New York: Springer Verlag; 1980.

Bransford JD, Brown AL, Cocking RR, eds. How people learn: brain, mind, experience, and school. Washington, DC: National Academy Press, 2000.

David T, Patel L, Burdett K, et al. Problem-based learning in medicine: a practical guide for students and teachers. London: The Royal Society of Medicine Press Ltd; 1999.

Hunter D, Bailey A, Taylor B. The art of facilitation. Auckland: Tandem Press; 2002.

Schwartz P, Mennin S, Webb G, eds. Problem-based learning: case studies, experience, practice. London: Kogan Page; 2001.

Wilkerson L, Gijselaers WH. Bringing problem-based learning to higher education: theory and practice. New directions for teaching and learning, No 68. San Francisco: Jossey-Bass; 1996.

ARTICLES AND RESEARCH PAPERS

Hmelo-Silver CE, Barrows HS. Goals and strategies of a problem-based learning facilitator. Interdiscip J Problem-based Learn 2006; 1(1):21–39.

Kamin C, O'Sullivan P, Deterding R, et al. A comparison of critical thinking in groups of third-year medical students in text, video, and virtual PBL case modalities. Acad Med 2003; 78(2):204–211.

Maudsley G. Do we all mean the same thing by "problem-based learning"? A review of the concepts and a formulation of the ground rules. Acad Med 1999; 74(2):178–185.

Roberts D, Ousey K. Problem based learning: developing the triggers. Experiences from a first wave site. Nurse Ed Prac 2003; 4(3): 154–158.

Schaber PL. Incorporating problem-based learning and video technology in teaching group process in an occupational therapy curriculum. J Allied Health 2005; 34(2):110–116.

Willis SC, Jones A, Bundy C, et al. Small-group work and assessment in a PBL curriculum: a qualitative and quantitative evaluation of student perceptions of the process of working in small groups and its assessment. Med Teach 2002; 24(5):494–501.

CHAPTER 3

Problem-based learning tutorials

I know [that] ... to do something well is to enjoy it.

PEARL S BUCK

INTRODUCTION

What is your perception of problem-based learning (PBL) tutorials?
How could you assess your own contribution in PBL tutorials?
What are the keys for success in PBL tutorials?

Over the last 15 years I have met hundreds of university students and helped a good number of them to achieve their goals and turn their challenges into opportunities for success. Many of them were first-year students and they came to see me 5 to 6 weeks after their enrolment. They were unable to find useful answers to the questions I've listed above and were not happy with their contribution in their PBL groups.

Likewise, you might be facing similar challenges. You may be coming from a school system in which you memorised factual material. You may have used your own private tutor to help you study different subjects and achieve high scores in examinations. Some of the students whom I helped used to learn from summaries, diagrams or tables prepared for them by a private tutor.

However, when they began at university they faced several challenges. They felt that they were not prepared for university education; that school had not prepared them for their new environment. They were used to being handed information and focusing only on factual knowledge. But learning at university requires cognitive skills, self-directed learning, application of knowledge, effective communication and interpersonal skills. In addition, in a PBL curriculum, students need these skills: the ability to deal with uncertainty, generate hypotheses, develop an enquiry plan, integrate knowledge from basic and clinical sciences, identify learning issues, use resources to construct new information, interpret the results of investigations and apply the knowledge learnt.

It is never too late to work out how to adopt a learning approach that suits the PBL structure and the university system. The challenge is not a result of the move to a different system. The real challenge lies in your perception of the new system and how you apply your skills and abilities to the system. In this chapter we will learn how to improve our contribution in PBL tutorials and the secrets for successful discussion of PBL cases.

ACTION VERBS

I hear, and I forget.
I read, and I remember.
I do, and I understand.

CHINESE PROVERB

What 'action verbs' dominate your PBL tutorials?

Action verbs specify what each member of the group is doing at a particular moment. They give you a good idea of the level of interaction in the group and the cognitive skills demonstrated as the group discusses the case. In my research into PBL, I have collected over 200 action verbs used by students. I have used these verbs in my research work to assess the effectiveness of PBL groups, the quality of contribution from members and to evaluate a number of learning strategies that can be used to improve student skills in PBL tutorials.

Action verbs can help you assess your own contribution to the group discussion and what areas you need to improve. In addition, you can use these verbs to enhance your own learning and develop the skills you need in a PBL curriculum. The essential action verbs are listed in the table on p. 36.

Before we start using this tool, I would like you to go through the table and read all the action verbs and think about each of them. This might take you 5–7 minutes.

Now read the following instructions:

- Before using the table make 12 copies and keep them for future reference.
- Using a green texta, highlight each action (verb) that you believe represents what you usually do in PBL tutorials.
- Using a red texta, highlight the actions you are *not* doing.
- Using a yellow texta, highlight actions you sometimes use but which you believe you are not using as much as you should.
- Write the date at the top of the page when you finish. Each day before you start your study, read the actions highlighted in red and yellow.
- Think about how using these actions could help expand your learning.
- After 2 weeks of continuous daily use of the list, start a new list on one of the other copies. With the same colours as above highlight the actions you are now using.
- When you finish, compare with your original list and observe your progress.
- Write down what you have achieved in 4 weeks and what strategies you could use to improve your skills.
- Keep doing this on a daily basis, starting a new list every 2 weeks. Keep the records in a folder.
- After 6 months, review your achievements. You will be astonished by the dramatic improvement in your learning skills, the quality of your contribution to your group and your deep understanding of the issues you are dealing with.

The evidence from my observations is that PBL groups which use these actions in their discussion at an optimal level are:

- focused on their learning outcomes
- able to demonstrate deep understanding of the concepts discussed
- getting the best out of each case
- engaged in their learning and believe that PBL enhances their learning.

DATE:

Semester:

Abstract	Define	Improve	Recognise
Achieve	Demonstrate	Inform	Record
Act	Describe	Initialise	Refine
Aim	Design	Innovate	Reflect
Analyse	Determine	Inspire	Register
Apply	Develop	Integrate	Rehearse
Ask questions	Differentiate	Internalise	Remember
Assess	Discover	Interpret	Research
Associate	Discuss	Investigate	Respond
Balance	Draw	Justify	Retrieve
Brainstorm	Edit	Label	Scan
Build mechanism	Elaborate	Lead	Scribe
Calculate	Eliminate	Learn	Search
Categorise	Encode	Listen	Select
Change	Encourage	Locate	Serve
Check	Energise	Manage	Set up
Clarify	Engage	Map	Share ideas
Classify	Enhance	Match	Show
Collaborate	Evaluate	Monitor	Solve
Collect	Examine	Motivate	Substitute
Collect data	Execute	Negotiate	Summarise
Communicate	Expand	Observe	Suppose
Compare	Experience	Organise	Synthesise
Compile	Explain	Perform	Target
Comprehend	Explore	Plan	Test
Concentrate	Extract	Point out	Think
Conceptualise	Facilitate	Practise	Transfer
Conclude	Familiarise	Predict	Understand
Consider	Finalise	Prepare	Undertake
Construct	Find out	Present	Upgrade
Construct tables	Function	Presume	Utilise
Convey	Gather	Process	Verify
Convince	Generate	Prove	Visualise
Coordinate	Group	Provide	Weigh evidence
Correct	Guide	Question	Work out
Create	Hypothesise	Rank	
Debate	Illustrate	Read	
Decide	Imagine	Reason	
	Implement	Receive	

GROUP MANAGEMENT, GROUP PROBLEMS

Some of the aims of learning in small groups include:
- achieving individual change and learning from other members
- valuing teamwork and collaborative learning
- fostering professional values, for example, effective communication, interpersonal skills, conflict resolution, showing respect for the views of others
- sharing ideas, learning from mistakes and from feedback
- understanding group organisation and group management
- developing skills in collaboration, not competition.

Effective group management, which helps achieve these aims, incorporates:
- identifying the group's ground rules and listing them on the whiteboard
- understanding the different roles each member could take on in a PBL tutorial, for example, scribe on the whiteboard, reader for the group, searching the resources and timing the group when working on a task
- allocating these roles
- discussing feedback and evaluating group function on a weekly basis. Members could commit the last 10 or 15 minutes for this purpose during which they raise questions such as: 'How is our group doing?' 'What are the areas we need to improve?' 'Did we use the time allocated to discuss each part of the case effectively?' 'Did we discuss the case to the depth needed?' Such discussion encourages members to come up with new ideas which they can put into effect as they work on a new case in the next week
- building a healthy environment in the group that accepts different views and gives everyone the opportunity to contribute.

These measures should be put in place when the group starts operating. However, problems may still appear and should be dealt with as they arise. Table 3.1 summarises sources of the problems and the symptoms associated with each.

Most problems are the result of the lack of the essential components for effective group function. As with a lack of vitamins in the human body, the group will present with a number of symptoms as a result of a particular deficiency. If you experience these symptoms in your group, it might be useful to share your thoughts with the group. You might make use of the weekly feedback session. Listen to other members' views and explore their perception. Agree on the causes of the problem, what is lacking, and what you need to do as a group to fix the problems.

QUALITIES OF A SUCCESSFUL GROUP

A successful PBL group will have the following characteristics:
- ground rules established by members when they start their first tutorial
- each member aware of their role
- members encouraged and motivated to achieve shared goals
- members focused on their tasks and using tutorial time effectively
- a tutor who has initiated a healthy and secure environment and who encourages the group to maintain this environment
- a tutor who has established trust and encouraged bonding of group members
- a tutor who acts as a role model for the group
- effective listening and effective communication

TABLE 3.1 Causes and symptoms of group dysfunction

Cause	Symptoms
1 Lack of ground rules	— More than one student talks at a time. — Members argue rather than debate issues. — When there are differences in views, members tend not to show respect for other members' views. — Not all members are involved in the discussion—one or two students dominate the group work.
2 Scribe on the whiteboard not appointed	— Group members repeat what was discussed. — Because members cannot see a list of hypotheses they find it difficult to refine their hypotheses or rank them. — Members find it difficult to follow through with what was discussed.
3 Absence of deep learning	— Groups leave tutorial rooms 30–45 minutes before the designated closing time. — Members use shortcuts in their discussion. — Members focus on diagnosis rather than discussion of the important concepts related to the case. — Members focus on factual knowledge rather than cognitive skills such as weighing evidence, justifying, comparing, collecting new information, building mechanisms. — Members do not use tables, flow diagrams or mechanisms to deepen their understanding of issues raised in the case.
4 Lack of teamwork	— Members do not share responsibility. — One or two students dominate the discussion. — Struggle between members creates an unhealthy group environment. — Members are not clear about their roles. — The decisions made are not discussed.
5 Poor time management	— Members spend too much time on the case discussion and find it difficult to complete the whole case in the assigned tutorial time. — Important tasks are not completed or are addressed briefly. — Members spend a lot of time on one specific issue; they are unable to find a balance between the big picture and fine details. — Members are slow in their discussion. — The tutorial usually starts 10–15 minutes late. — Members do not allocate time to complete a task before they commence working on it.
6 Poor facilitation	— Members find it difficult to discuss new and difficult concepts. — There are gaps in their discussion and they tend to take shortcuts. — Members are not interested in the discussion. — Members are not engaged and are unsure of the benefits of PBL tutorials.
7 Lack of focus	— Members spend too much time on peripheral issues. — Members are not able to identify their priorities. — Members do not focus on key issues raised in the case. — Members are not clear about their roles.
8 Ineffective communication	— Members lack listening skills. — Members do not build upon what was discussed. — Discussion at times seems to be meaningless. — Members at times struggle in their communication and conflict may become apparent.

TABLE 3.1 Causes and symptoms of group dysfunction *continued*

Cause	Symptoms
9 Absence of deep understanding	— Members focus on factual knowledge. — Members fail to identify several important learning issues related to the case. — Members confuse knowledge and become unsure. — Discussion lacks integration of knowledge and lateral and critical thinking. — Members do not use open-ended questions to deepen their discussion.
10 Poor motivation	— A spirit of competition rather than collaboration dominates the group. — Not everyone contributes to the discussion. — Members are not interested in PBL, they arrive late and the discussion is usually slow or they use shortcuts. — Members are not engaged or creative in the way they work together. — Members treat the PBL tutorial simply as routine work.

- feedback used to rise to new challenges
- members able to resolve conflict and deal with problems as they emerge
- members using evidence in making decisions
- no favouritism or bias.

KEYS FOR SUCCESSFUL GROUP DISCUSSION

How can your group develop these characteristics?

Although successful discussion of a PBL case in a tutorial has been attributed to several factors, including authenticity of the case, flow and design of the case, and skills of the PBL tutor, the real key for a successful PBL discussion remains in the hands of the students who should be oriented to the philosophy of problem-based learning, the rationale for its use and their role in a tutorial (see Chs 1 and 2).

Here are twelve practical ways to help you discuss a PBL case with your group in a successful manner. They will help your group overcome the problems observed in some PBL groups and reported in the literature.

→ KEY 1 MAINTAIN GROUND RULES

- Ground rules (group norms) are set early in a group's existence to prevent dysfunction and are agreed upon by group members.
- They should reflect on the group's needs and principles.
- The tutor should discuss their role with the group.
- Groups should operate according to the rules.

Here are some examples of ground rules defined by a PBL group:
- Everyone has the right to express their view.
- We should debate issues rather than argue them.
- We should not spend too much time on one issue.
- We should respect each other and avoid personal comments.
- We need one scribe at a time—two (or even three) scribes per tutorial.
- We need a recorder for each tutorial.
- We need to focus on the discussion of the case and avoid getting side-tracked.

Some of the ground rules are non-negotiable as they are important for group function and will be explained by your tutor:
- Attendance and punctuality are mandatory.
- All mobile phones must be turned off during the tutorial.
- Groups must use the whiteboard as they discuss the case.
- The case should be discussed in the outlined sequence.
- The group should not take shortcuts or skip a step.

What to do if ground rules are ignored
Here are some suggestions:
- Explain why you believe it is important that ground rules are followed (development of group autonomy, prevention of group dysfunction, enhancement of group dynamics, allowing everyone to have their turn).
- Provide solutions that can help your group grow.
- Talk with passion about your views. Be clear and firm about each point.
- Do not argue with people who do not agree with you.
- If your initiatives do not work, do not give up. Outside the tutorials talk with group members about group organisation, group dynamics and ground rules.
- Talk to your tutor at the end of the tutorial.
- Remember that positive messages are contagious.
- Choose a paper from the literature related to this issue, provide a copy to your tutor and ask them if the group can debate the benefits of ground rules. Timing is very important: your suggestions may be more acceptable if raised after a struggle or a problem in the group caused by the lack of ground rules.

➔ KEY 2 KNOW YOUR ROLES

- Groups function best when each member is aware of the different roles.
- Roles should be agreed upon and organised in the first tutorial of a block/semester.

   What are the roles available to you in a PBL tutorial?

- *Be a scribe*: a scribe listens to each member's input, records and organises information discussed by the group on the whiteboard, encourages every member to contribute and knows how to serve the group. It might be useful to have three scribes in a two-hour tutorial, each one scribing for about 40 minutes.
- *Be involved in the case discussion*: every member contributes to the discussion in a way that adds new information, deepens group understanding, acknowledges others' input, focuses on the issue and avoids negative arguments.
- *Be a group recorder* (on paper): a group recorder summarises all the information on the whiteboard and makes a hard copy available to each member after the tutorial.
- *Be a word finder*: look up difficult terms in the medical dictionary.
- *Be the group's representative*: each semester, one member is nominated by the group to represent them at faculty meetings and look after administrative issues in the group.

   Apart from the group's representative, students rotate roles every tutorial. A student may have more than one role in the same tutorial.

What to do if two or three members dominate
This is a common problem in groups that have failed to define the ground rules and specify the role of each member in the group.
- Addressing this problem in the group at an early stage is important, but it is never too late to solve problems in the group.
- Do not wait for others to raise their concerns.
- If you feel that you do not have the courage to 'blow the whistle', talk to your tutor in private about your concerns. Ask them to mention in the next tutorial that some group members have raised issues they feel the group needs to discuss and that they wish to clarify the role of each member. This initiative may help other students in the group to speak out.
- The group should discuss the distribution of roles and the use of a mechanism that allows each member to play an active role in the group. Sometimes one or two members in the group will decline to take on their role. The tutor may discuss this with those students when they provide feedback to each member of the group.

→ KEY 3 FOSTER GROUP DYNAMICS

- Ask yourself: What good qualities am I bringing to my group?
- Use individual and cultural differences as a way to foster group dynamics.
- Appreciate the value of teamwork and the need for regular evaluation of the group process.
- The last 10 minutes in tutorial 2 (as you complete the discussion of a case) are a good opportunity for the group to reflect on members' performance, identify specific goals that the group aims for and plan how to achieve each of these goals. Focus on one goal at a time.

Group performance review: what are the questions to ask?
- What did we achieve this week as a group?
- Have we worked together effectively?
- In what areas did we succeed?
- In what areas do we need improvement?
- As a group, what are our goals for next week?
- What mechanisms will we use to achieve these goals?

Main differences between effective and dysfunctional groups

Effective groups	Dysfunctional groups
Maintain their ground rules	Fail to identify ground rules
Members focus on group's goals	Members do not have common goals
Care about team achievements	Care about personal gains
Work in a supportive environment	Tutor-centred or managed by a dominant student
Regularly discuss strategies to improve their performance	Satisfied with their performance
Give priority to continuous group monitoring	Ignore feedback

→ KEY 4 ASK EMPOWERING QUESTIONS

- Use good open-ended questions to improve discussion and keep the group focused on the issue.
- Using empowering questions in a group discussion is vital for deep understanding and better learning.
- Avoid asking shallow questions that focus on detail.
  Examples of open-ended questions that enhance group discussion of a case:
- Normally we do not feel short of breath. What structures and functions do we need so that we breathe normally?
- What could go wrong with each of these structures and cause shortness of breath?
- What are the structures in the chest that could cause chest pain?
- What could go wrong with each of these structures and cause chest pain?

What are the purposes of questioning?
Good open-ended questions help learners to:
- participate actively in the discussion
- think, reflect, link information and make priorities
- discuss divergent opinions
- highlight important concepts and deepen their understanding
- assess other aspects of a concept
- focus on what they are doing and make the discussion purposeful.

→ KEY 5 BE A PURPOSEFUL LEARNER

- A powerful motivator for learning is keeping the learning process purposeful so that it contributes to personal growth and deep understanding.
- Your self-directed learning will be enhanced if you know exactly what questions you are trying to answer in your search.
- Shape your learning to suit the needs of your new learning environment.

  A purposeful learner:
- has a continuous desire for knowledge
- is focused on their goals
- is a critical thinker
- is self-motivated
- is not afraid to ask for help
- is able to monitor their own progress
- has an enquiry plan
- is able to integrate information learnt
- has developed reasoning skills
- plans their learning
- strives for excellence
- is eager to receive feedback
- is aware of their strengths and weaknesses.

As a learner, what strategies do you use to empower yourself?
- Focus on goals and outcomes.
- Encourage and motivate people working with you, not just yourself.
- Get in to the habit of positive thinking.
- Become a purpose-driven person.
- Enjoy what you are learning.

→ KEY 6 WITHOUT FEEDBACK THERE WOULD BE NO CHAMPIONS

- Learn how to get the best out of your tutor's feedback.
- With your tutor, plan how to use feedback to enhance your input to the group discussion and boost your learning.

  What are the characteristics of good feedback?
  Good feedback is:
- clear
- given immediately
- descriptive, not judgemental
- specific rather than general
- directed at a person's behaviour rather than at the person
- both positive and negative
- delivered in a climate of trust and collaboration
- negotiated rather than imposed.

How can you benefit most from your tutor's feedback?
- Focus on the issues raised in the feedback and don't take it personally.
- Show interest in the issues raised and explore them with your tutor.
- Negotiate an approach with your tutor to enhance your input to the group.
- Work on one issue at a time and meet with your tutor in a fortnight to discuss your progress.
- Think about ways to keep yourself motivated and continuously improving.
- Keep monitoring yourself and focus on your goals.
- Record your daily progress in a journal.
- Once you have accomplished a particular skill, move on to the next area in need of improvement.
- Celebrate your successes.

→ KEY 7 MONITOR YOUR PROGRESS

- One of the key elements of success is self-evaluation and motivation.
- Keep focused on your goals as you progress.
- Keep a journal to monitor your progress.

What issues should you address in your progress journal?
- What are my areas of strength?
- What are the skills I am still developing?
- What are the skills I need to improve?　　　　　　　　　　→

- How can I improve myself in each of these areas?
- Do I need help from my tutor?
- What type of help do I need?
- How can I learn from my group members?
- What are my priorities?

→ KEY 8 STRIVE TO BE A WINNING TEAM

- Effective interactions fuel the right actions.
- Focus on the issue rather than personal interest.
- Group success is the outcome of every member's contribution and commitment.
- Think positively about others in your group.

    Characteristics of winning teams:
- They define their priorities effectively.
- They give up their personal plans when required.
- They appreciate the process of developing people.
- They communicate effectively.
- They encourage team membership.
- They establish their common goals.
- They are committed to the group.

How can you help build your group?
- Be an encourager.
- Accept other members in your group and show interest in everyone.
- Invest in working with others.
- Be positive and constructive in your views.
- Establish effective links with other members.
- Focus on group achievements rather than on personal gains.
- Share your resources with others.
- To be a good leader serve other members and enjoy working with the team.
- Be open to criticism.
- Think about ways of enhancing group function.
- Maintain your commitment to the group work.

→ KEY 9 BE A CRITICAL THINKER

- Debate rather than argue an issue.
- Before making decisions, weigh evidence for and against an hypothesis.
    Characteristics of critical thinkers:
- Use their thinking abilities to the fullest extent. For example, they keep asking questions and explore different aspects of a new issue.
- Carefully analyse complex issues.
- Develop a thoughtful and well-structured approach to guide their choices.
- Look for supportive evidence for each of their hypotheses.
- Evaluate data, synthesise information, establish links and identify areas that need further research.
- Able to discuss issues in an organised fashion that shows logical or sequential flow.

- Evaluate the accuracy of their beliefs.
- Have a passion for understanding and always strive to solve problems.
- Explore different aspects of an issue, for example, scientific basis, ethical and moral issues, background and contributing factors.

How can you debate issues rather than argue them?
We *debate* issues when we discuss them with no or minimal personal bias, whereas when we *argue* them we bring our personal bias into the argument and we tend to ignore the views of others.
- Always think about solutions that can help your group grow.
- Ask yourself first whether the point you raise will be of any significance to the current discussion.
- Focus your discussion on the issue itself and be objective.
- Avoid personal attacks.
- Explain your views and be clear.
- Leave the group members to further reflect on what was said.
- Accept other members' views and be flexible.
- Remember that the main aim is to help the group discussion rather than to achieve personal goals.

→ KEY 10 UNDERSTAND YOUR TUTOR'S ROLE

- The approach in PBL is student-centred.
- Your tutor will not be the information provider.
- Your tutor will facilitate learning and put the discussion on the right track when needed.
- During one-on-one sessions, your tutor will provide you with feedback on your contribution to group discussion.
- Your tutor will provide the group with the opportunity to discuss ways of improving group dynamics when you finish the discussion of each problem.

Knowing the role of your tutor in a PBL course, what does this mean to you?
- I need to be more active in my learning approach.
- I have the responsibility to work effectively with my group members.
- I should trust the student–centred approach as a way of learning.
- I should participate in the group discussion and understand my roles in the tutorial.

How does the tutor's role differ in PBL and traditional learning?
- The PBL tutor is a facilitator. In a traditional course they provide information.
- The PBL tutor fosters collaborative learning. In a traditional course they foster one-way learning.
- The PBL tutor encourages critical thinking. In a traditional course they foster the acquisition of factual knowledge.
- The PBL tutor is not necessarily an expert in the subject matter. In a traditional course they must be a content resource.
- The PBL tutor focuses on the students' needs and the group discussion. In a traditional course they focus on what they want to teach.
- The PBL tutor monitors the group discussion. In a traditional course they direct the whole session. ➡

- The PBL tutor asks open-ended questions at times. In a traditional course they ask and answer all questions.
- The PBL tutor listens carefully to the group interaction. In a traditional course they speak throughout the session.
- The PBL tutor enhances the learning process and models the various steps of the reasoning process. In a traditional course they emphasise the memorising of information.
- The PBL tutor is a mentor, motivator and feedback provider. In a traditional course they are a knowledge deliverer.

→ KEY 11 DEVELOP A WINNING ATTITUDE

- Develop good habits.
- Select a model to follow.
- See opportunities for success in challenges.
- Focus on solutions.
- Have a desire to give and share resources.
- Be persistent.
- Find ways to relieve stress.
- Don't take yourself too seriously.
- Take action to change your attitude.

How can you become part of a productive team?
- Share resources with other students in your group.
- Share the information you collect with others.
- Think about the group progress and your contribution to this process.
- Discuss the best options to enhance group dynamics with group members.

→ KEY 12 BE A COLLABORATIVE LEARNER

Collaboration is the critical competency for achieving and improving group performance. To foster collaboration group members should:
- create a climate of trust
- ask others for help when needed
- listen attentively to the views of other members
- interact with each other on a regular basis
- share information and resources
- provide descriptive rather than evaluative or judgemental comments
- ask questions for clarification
- always say 'we'.

Why is collaborative learning useful?
- It allows learners to share their views and experiences.
- It allows learners to evaluate what they have learnt and develop new skills.
- It motivates students to improve their performance.
- Research has shown that information acquired via collaborative learning is better retained in the long-term memory compared to information learnt from reading a textbook or listening to a lecture.

THE SEVEN RULES OF PROBLEM-BASED LEARNING

Questions that are commonly heard from first-year students enrolled in PBL courses include:

- Do I need to change my learning style?
- How can I create this new learning style?
- What should I do to enhance my learning?
- I prefer to stay as I am, but I do not feel that I am doing well despite long hours of learning. How can I be sure that I am using an effective style of learning?
- Do I need to remember everything in the textbook?

I am sure that you also have similar questions. The seven rules listed here provide answers in a nutshell. See Chs 4 to 9 for detailed answers.

Rule 1: There is no ideal way to learn but you need to change your learning style to suit the needs of the PBL curriculum.

Rule 2: Change your learning style by focusing on deep understanding rather than memorising information.

Rule 3: Deepen your learning by targeting these skills:

- integrating information learnt from several resources
- assessing the different aspects of a newly learnt concept
- applying the knowledge learnt to real-life situations
- looking for supportive evidence and assessing the level of evidence
- linking the new information learnt to what is already known
- identifying areas of deficiencies in what is learnt and planning to search for more information
- using educational tools such as tables, flow diagrams or illustrations to outline the new information
- presenting information learnt to others in a clear and comprehensive manner using your own learning style.

Rule 4: Be a critical thinker. Learning is an active process and you need to be motivated to look for new information which will answer your questions.

Rule 5: Never be satisfied with what you have learnt. Do not swim near the shore; go into deep waters.

Rule 6: Take responsibility for your own learning. What I mean here is that the whole process is yours and you have to take ownership and always be in control. See the differences between students who are responsible for their learning and those who avoid responsibility (Table 3.2).

Rule 7: Monitor your progress. Keep looking for ways to improve your learning skills and foster your ability to use and apply the information learnt.

CONCLUSIONS

In PBL, students work in small groups in a collaborative way to solve real-life problems. In this process, students learn content and expand their higher-order thinking and communication skills. For successful discussion of PBL cases, students need to change their learning style to suit the needs of PBL. They need to understand the educational objectives of PBL, the rationale for using PBL, the problems they may encounter in PBL tutorials, the qualities of successful group discussion and the keys for successful discussion of a case. By using the keys for success discussed in this chapter you will develop a clear idea of your roles in a PBL tutorial and how to make the most of each of those roles.

TABLE 3.2 Student responsibility for learning: acceptance and avoidance

Students taking full responsibility for their learning	Students avoiding responsibility for their learning
Are always in full control	Feel helpless and not in control
Accept responsibility for their actions	Deny responsibility when they perform badly
Have a consistent approach to their learning	Do not have a specific style or approach to their learning
Always monitor their progress and look for new skills to acquire	Cannot acquire new skills
Focus on solutions when they face challenges	Blame circumstances, teachers, the school when they face challenges
Choose to study and enjoy learning	Feel that learning is a duty
Keep empowering and motivating themselves	Miss out on improving their skills. Feel they are not learning, despite spending long hours reading
Learn from their mistakes	Try to cover up and ignore their mistakes
Know what they need to learn and how	Are not sure of what they need to learn or how to do so
Are able to express their learning needs by: — asking questions — participating in class discussions — learning to fulfil their own needs — sharing information with others	Do not express themselves well by: — declining to ask questions — avoiding participation in discussion — learning routinely — preferring to listen

EVIDENCE-BASED LEARNING
Student perspectives on learning-oriented interactions in the tutorial group

This is a recent study from Maastricht University, the Netherlands, where the researchers used a questionnaire to measure students' perceptions of occurrence and desirability of three interaction types: (1) exploratory questioning, (2) cumulative reasoning, and (3) handling knowledge conflicts. The discrepancies between the perceptions of occurrence and desirability enabled the researchers to illustrate how the questionnaire can be used to improve the group interaction process in PBL tutorials. The study comprised all second-year medical students (n = 240, response rate 73%). The questionnaire consisted of a list of 11 statements representing the three interaction types (factors). Students were asked to rate each statement on a 5-point Likert scale for two types of perceptions, that is, occurrence and desirability. The results show that average scores on occurrence and desirability of the interaction types varied between 3.4 and 3.7 (scale 1–5) and between 3.6 and 4.3, respectively. For two interaction types, significant differences between occurrence and desirability were found. The researchers concluded that the scores for occurrence were reasonable, and the desirability scores were significantly higher than the occurrence scores for two of the three interaction types, that is, exploratory questioning and cumulative reasoning. The results of the study imply that in the students' opinion, the interaction process in the tutorial group can be improved

The questionnaire used in the study provides useful information to detect shortcomings in tutorial group interaction.

Visschers-Pleijers AJ, Dolmans DH, Ineke HA, et al. Adv Health Sci Educ Theory Prac 2005; 10(1):23–35. Adapted with permission from the publisher.
For more information: http://www.springerlink.com/content/1573-1677/

FURTHER READING
BOOKS
David T, Patel L, Burdett K, et al. Problem-based learning in medicine: a practical guide for students and teachers. London: The Royal Society of Medicine Press Ltd; 1999.
Barrows HS. Problem-based learning applied to medical education. Rev edn. Springfield, Ill: Southern Illinois University School of Medicine; 2000.

ARTICLES AND RESEARCH PAPERS
Azer SA. Becoming a student in a PBL course: twelve tips for successful group discussion. Med Teach 2004; 26(1):12–15.
Azer SA. Challenges facing PBL tutors: 12 tips for successful group facilitation. Med Teach 2005; 27(8):676–681.
Blumberg P, Michael JA, Zeitz H. Roles of student-generated learning issues in problem-based learning. Teach Learn Med 1990; 2(3):149–154.
Burns ER. Learning syndromes afflicting beginning medical students: identification and treatment—reflections after forty years of teaching. Med Teach 2006; 28(3):230–233.
Charlin B, Mann K, Hansen P. The many faces of problem-based learning: a framework for understanding and comparison. Med Teach 1998; 20(4):323 330.

Chaves JF, Lantz MS, Lynch MD. Tutor and student perceptions of the tutor's role in problem-based learning. J Dent Educ 2001; 65(3):222–230.

Das M, Mpofu DJ, Hasan MY, et al. Student perceptions of tutor skills in problem-based learning tutorials. Med Educ 2002; 36(3):272–278.

Dolmans DH, Schmidt HG. What do we know about cognitive and motivational effects of small group tutorials in problem-based learning? Adv Health Sci Theory Prac 2006; 11(4):321–336.

Gilkison A. Techniques used by "expert" and "non-expert" tutors to facilitate problem-based learning tutorials in undergraduate medical curriculum. Med Educ 2003; 37(1):6–14.

Hmelo-Silver CE. Problem-based learning: What and how do students learn? Educ Psychol Review 2004; 16:235–266.

Kaufman DM, Holmes DB. Tutoring in problem-based learning: perceptions of teachers and students. Med Educ 1996; 30(5):371–377.

Maudsley G. Roles and responsibilities of the problem-based learning tutor in the undergraduate medical curriculum. BMJ 1999; 318(7184):657–661.

Neville AJ. The problem-based learning tutor: Teacher? Facilitator? Evaluator? Med Teach 1999; 21(4):394–401.

Ravens U, Nitsche I, Haag C, et al. What is a good tutorial from the student's point of view? Evaluation of tutorials in a newly established PBL block course "Basics of Drug Therapy". Naunyn-Schmiedeberg's Archives Pharmacol 2002; 366 (1):69–76.

Visschers-Pleijers AJ, Dolmans DH, Wolfhagen IH, et al. Student perspectives on learning-oriented interactions in the tutorial group. Adv Health Sci Educ Theory Prac 2005; 10(1):23–35.

PART TWO

STUDY SKILLS IN PROBLEM-BASED LEARNING

CHAPTER 4

Self-directed learning

If physicians would read two articles per day out of the six million medical articles published annually, in one year, they would fall 82 centuries behind in their reading   **WILLIAM F MISER**

INTRODUCTION

With the introduction of problem-based learning (PBL) in medical and health professional curricula, self-directed learning (also known as self-regulated learning) becomes an integral component of the learning process. There may be variations in how educators define self-directed learning; the following conceptual framework provides a clear definition and outlines its objectives:

* The learner is autonomous and able to articulate their learning needs, identify their goals, differentiate these into a number of objectives and able to decide on the learning resources needed for their learning. They are also able to construct new information and evaluate the quality of their own learning.
* The learner assumes primary control at specific stages.
* As a result, the learner develops the personal qualities and attributes to become an independent learner and is able to use this new learning process to further their personal development.
* Self-directed learning has a lifelong perspective. It is not just limited to adult learning.

Self-directed learning provides an opportunity for collaborative discussion of new information collected and allows learners to construct the information as they address their learning issues. It is not just about searching for new knowledge; it is also about developing competencies, skills and attitudes that foster the learning process.

I do not think that all learners are able to take up this way of learning immediately they enrol in a PBL curriculum. The process is gradual. As a learner you should:

* realise the need to change your learning style to suit the needs of the PBL curriculum
* construct a plan to accommodate your new learning objectives
* practise self-directed learning and share your experiences with your peers
* continually evaluate your self-directed learning approach.

The aim of this chapter is not to provide you with the theories behind self-directed learning or the research outcomes in this area. My aim is to encourage you to:

* understand the meaning of self-directed learning in the context of PBL
* understand the different factors that may affect your self-directed learning
* learn how to develop your self-directed learning skills by applying 12 keys that help you practise and develop these skills.

TRADITIONAL AND SELF-DIRECTED LEARNING: A COMPARISON

The traditional learning process is characterised by didactic instruction where information is presented by the teacher to the students. Teaching is usually delivered to a large group of students and the teacher is the sole provider of information. Students may ask questions at the end of the lesson. However, they are not engaged in a way that encourages them to think about the information provided, generate hypotheses, consider possible contributing factors or causes of a problem, search for information, weigh evidence, construct a plan, make decisions or deal with uncertainty.

In self-directed learning students are in control of their learning: they identify their learning needs, look for resources, search for new information and construct the information that answers their learning objectives. Self-directed learning also develops a wide range of skills and competencies, not just those of identifying knowledge or finding answers. PBL curricula provide excellent opportunities for learners to develop their self-directed learning. Table 4.1 summarises the main differences between traditional and self-directed learning in a PBL environment.

How can PBL enhance self-directed learning?
- PBL is a student-centred approach
- Students use cases in their learning and discussion questions aimed at improving cognitive skills and deep understanding.
- Students discuss cases with minimal or no knowledge about the case.
- Teachers in PBL are facilitators rather than information providers.
- In PBL, students need to identify their own learning needs.

In the self-directed environment of a PBL curriculum students need to:
- use learning issues as the basis for their search
- use a number of resources in different disciplines at the same time
- construct information from several resources rather than copy or summarise what they have read
- search for answers to their questions rather than memorising a chapter or a lecture
- integrate information across disciplines and see relationships, for example, (1) identify structural functional relationships; (2) examine how their knowledge of physiology can help them understand the mechanisms by which drugs work, the pathogenesis of the disease and the factors contributing to malfunction; and (3) examine relationships between clinical medicine and basic sciences
- use information learnt to interpret the patient's laboratory findings, explain the scientific basis for the patient's signs and symptoms, provide justifications, weigh evidence for and against each hypothesis generated as well as create a mechanism (e.g. a flow chart) to summarise the patient's problems and its pathogenesis
- be ready to share in group discussion and contribute to collaborative learning
- be ready to debate issues raised in group discussion in tutorial 2
- apply the information collected in tutorial 2, the remaining two or three progress stages and the closure of the case.
- demonstrate the ability to be an active learner in the group: clarifying issues, asking good questions, and adding to what others in the group have identified.

WHY DEVELOP SELF-DIRECTED SKILLS?

The quote from Miser at the start of this chapter clearly describes the impact of the rapid explosion of research publications in the past 10 to 15 years. With the reduction

TABLE 4.1 Main differences between problem-based and traditional learning

Problem-based learning	Traditional learning
Students learn in small groups	Students learn in large groups
Student-centred approach	Teacher-centred approach
Focus is on learning, developing skills and competencies	Focus is on information
Students are engaged in the discussion for 2 hours per session	Students often lose concentration after 10–15 minutes
Strong and continuous interaction between students	No interaction between students
Learning is mainly based on collaborative learning	It is a one-person show (the teacher's)
Students learn from their mistakes and misunderstandings	No opportunity for learning from mistakes and misunderstandings
Class is driven by students	Class is driven by teacher
Learning is focused on cognitive skills, such as: — integration of knowledge — generating hypotheses — searching for information — weighing the evidence — interpreting findings	Learning is focused on: — regurgitation of information — subject content
Role of teacher is to facilitate discussion	Role of teacher is to transmit ideas and knowledge
The focus is on application of knowledge	The focus is on theories
Learners retain information in their long-term memory	Learners have poor retention of information learnt
Students are able to see relationships between issues learnt	Students often do not understand the relationships between issues
A wide range of resources are used by learners	Recommended textbooks are the main resources used

in the number of lectures and the requirement for students to discuss cases with no prior knowledge about case content and deal with the uncertainty this creates, the need for self-directed learning becomes essential. You should develop the skill of self-directed learning during your undergraduate years if you are to cope with the rapid explosion in research publications.

KEYS FOR IMPROVING YOUR SELF-DIRECTED LEARNING

Students I teach in PBL courses ask me questions such as, 'What are the methods we can use to improve our self-directed learning?' 'Are there any tips to foster our skills in this area?' 'We are still not sure whether our learning is going in the right direction. Is there any way to know?' 'How can we change our learning style?' and 'How can we achieve what we need through self-directed learning?'

From my reading and research I have developed 12 keys to help you develop your own self-directed model and adjust your learning style to meet the objectives of PBL. Read these keys and use your reflective journal to record the actions you will take with regard to each key. Putting these keys into an action plan when you start your PBL course will enable you to develop a competency model for your self-directed learning and to move ahead week by week.

→ KEY 1 CHANGE YOUR LEARNING STYLE

Why do you need to change your learning style?
- In problem–based learning courses the number of lectures is reduced.
- These lectures focus on the key principles and supply few details. They introduce concepts and engage you with questions you might need to address in your learning.
- The whole approach of learning in PBL is student-centred; the role of tutors is to facilitate discussion.
- You work on PBL cases so you need to search for new information to address the learning issues identified at the end of tutorial 1.
- The course is designed to give you the opportunity to search for information and apply the information learnt.
- In such courses, you need to develop a number of competencies and skills on your own.

How do you start the process of change?
- Think about the main differences between a traditional course you have done and a PBL curriculum.
- Think about why learning in a PBL curriculum necessitates a change in your learning approach.
- Think about the learning skills and competencies you need in a PBL curriculum.
- Write down the skills and competencies you possess and how you could use them to plan your new learning style.
- Give priority to this issue. Start working on it as you commence your course.
- Identify your learning needs.
- Remember it is your responsibility to make learning meaningful.
- Create a sense of ownership of what you plan to do and be passionate about the changes you will make.
- Use a reflective journal to address these questions and the rationale for your changes.

→ KEY 2 IDENTIFY YOUR LEARNING NEEDS

- A *learning need* is the gap between where you are and where you want to be with regard to achieving particular skills and competencies.
- You might become aware of these needs from personal feedback, past experiences or from daily work practices.
- The more clear you are about what you need, the more you will become aware of the gaps and the fine detail of what you need.
- The needs can include deficiencies in knowledge and attitudes, skills and competencies.

What questions should I ask to identify my learning needs?
- What do I know in this area?
- What do I need to achieve?
- What skills and competencies do I need to acquire?
- What else is stopping me from achieving in this area?
- In what way are any new needs related to my main needs?
- Am I clear about what I need? How can I build on my knowledge and experiences to fill the gap?

→ KEY 3 CONSTRUCT A LEARNING MODEL FOR COMPETENCIES

- Start with a beginning model of competencies you wish to acquire.
- Your model may include a number of skills such as (1) effective use of MEDLINE search; (2) new techniques to identify key questions related to the case; (3) using a textbook, journal articles and multimedia resources to construct new information; and (4) using new information to address issues raised in the case discussion.
- Your model may also include skills such as scribing in a PBL tutorial, communication skills and establishing rapport, evaluating your learning, testing your abilities and what you have accomplished.
- When you have determined what you know and what you do not yet know, you can develop a plan to guide your efforts in applying the model and achieving your goals over several months.

Your learning model may consist of these components:
- identifying areas of learning needs
- turning your learning needs into learning objectives
- identifying knowledge, skills and competencies needed for each objective
- identifying your learning resources
- planning your approach to use these resources and collect new information
- constructing new information, building mechanisms, designing tables, concept maps and diagrams
- preparing yourself for group discussion, revisiting what you have learnt and thinking about questions that may be raised and how you will handle them
- checking your resources again; you may need new resources to answer the new questions
- assessing how the new knowledge relates to what you already know and in what way it is related
- evaluating what you have learnt and your overall learning plan. Think about ways to improve your learning model.

PBL: a learning model for self-directed learning
Q 1:   What is your purpose? Why are you learning? What are you aiming for?
Q 2:   What did you learn in tutorial 1? What are the key principles raised in the case? Why did you study this case? Why did the faculty recommend this case for your learning?   ➡

Q 3:   If you want to summarise these key principles what will you say? What is the big picture in this case?

Q 4:   What are the learning issues identified by the group?

Q 5:   What are your learning objectives? What other questions could you think of for each learning issue? Do you have any other questions that can be related to these learning issues and explain what you really need to know?

Q 6:   What are the key resources you will use? Which resource would you start with?

Q 7:   What key information is important here?

Q 8:   Did this information answer your questions? What is missing? How can you summarise the information collected so far?

Q 9:   How can you organise this information? Would it be best to place the information in a table? What about using a flow chart? What about using a diagram?

Q 10:   How can you link the information learnt?

Q 11:   What analogy might you use for remembering this information? How can the clinical scenario help you to hook this information?

Q 12:   How can this new information link to what you have learnt previously?

Q 13:   What is your evaluation of what you learnt? How can you foster your learning for the next week? What are the things you need to change in your approach?

→ KEY 4 SPECIFY YOUR LEARNING OBJECTIVES

- Your learning objectives should describe what you will learn, not what you will do.
- Your learning objectives should define the learning needs you have identified as either competencies, skills, attitudes or values.
- Think about your priorities and the strategies you will use to achieve your goals.
- Specify target dates for completion of each task and the follow-up needed for each.
- Be realistic. Consider your learning needs, the curriculum structure and the time available to implement your plan.

  Examples of learning objectives:
- *Knowledge*: Acquiring new information, applying it to work out new problems, integrating it with what is already known, constructing new information from the resources used, testing the evidence provided and identifying deficiencies in the knowledge collected.
- *Understanding*: Interpreting laboratory results, providing justification, understanding the scientific basis for the patient's presenting symptoms and clinical signs.
- *Skills*: Asking good open-ended questions, creating a healthy environment when taking a history, developing communication skills, clinical examination skills and procedural skills.
- *Attitude*: Performance in real-life situations, role playing and simulation.
- *Values*: The ethical or moral issues that concern you in critical incident cases, decision-making and what values you bring to your practice.

What are the aims of learning objectives?
Learning objectives help learners to:
- identify what they want to learn: knowledge, skills, attitudes, values
- think, reflect, link information and make priorities
- discuss what they need to do
- highlight important concepts and deepen their understanding
- focus on what they want to learn.

How can I know that my objectives are adequately addressed?
The learning objectives should be:
- comprehensive
- up-to-date
- clear and precise
- authentic
- evidence-based
- useful
- able to provide answers to the questions raised
- deep and broad in their coverage
- logical in their flow
- applicable so learners can solve similar problems
- integrated
- able to be presented as flow charts, tables or other mechanisms
- able to provide explanations of the changes observed.

→ KEY 5 IDENTIFY LEARNING RESOURCES TO USE

What makes a good learning resource? It is:
- written for undergraduate students
- up-to-date, authentic and evidence-based
- designed to improve the learning process
- organised, easy to read, interactive, integrated and engaging
- designed to match with the philosophy of the curriculum.

A good learning resource also:
- covers theories and their practical applications
- uses tables, flow charts, diagrams, digital images and concept maps to explain complex issues
- contains chapters or modules that end with dot-point summaries, applications, review questions and scenario-based questions
- allows students to reflect on the main concepts learnt and to assess their learning skills.

As a learner, how could you use these learning resources effectively?
- Review the contents page and the organisation of each resource.
- Practise using each resource and how to get the most out of it.
- When you search for information, start with the resource that will provide you with the overall picture of your learning issues. Then use resources that will provide you with the detail of each issue. ➡

- Learn how to effectively use the tables, flow charts and diagrams provided in your resources.
- Learn how to integrate related information from two or three resources. For example, the answer to your question may come from several resources, each one of which provides you with a different reason.

→ KEY 6 PROVIDE EVIDENCE OF YOUR LEARNING ACHIEVEMENTS

- Learn how to measure your learning progress.
- Check the indicators for your learning performance and achievements.

  The evidence for learning achievements includes:
- degree of engagement in the group discussion
- performance and contribution to information constructed by the group
- learning new skills and demonstrating improvement in specific competencies
- becoming passionate about self-directed learning and efficient in time management
- increasing self confidence and the ability to handle challenging situations
- your learning portfolio records
- feedback from tutors, mentors and peers
- performance in the *formative assessment*
- performance in the *summative assessment* (see Glossary).

Why do learners need to measure their accomplishments?
Learners want to:
- know that they have accomplished a task and that they have achieved their objectives
- confirm what they have learnt
- identify gaps in their learning process
- improve their performance
- celebrate their success.

→ KEY 7 NEVER BE SATISFIED

- Get curious. Ask the five key questions: What? Where? When? Why? How?
- Dig deeper. Ask questions such as:
    —What if …?
    —What would happen if …?
    —What are the contributing factors?
    —What does this mean to me?
    —What are the uses of this information clinically?
    —What does this remind me of?
    —What knowledge is missing here?
- Consider your questions in order of significance to your learning and the case discussion.
- Develop a passion about what you are learning and creating.

What drives self-directed learning in a PBL curriculum?
The following factors drive self-directed learning:
- the nature and structure of the curriculum (e.g. students discuss problems in small groups without prior knowledge about the problems)
- tutors facilitating the group discussion and not providing information
- problems designed to engage students and allow them to raise questions and discuss issues
- facilitating questions enabling students to construct rich cognitive models of the concepts discussed
- a healthy group environment allowing each student to express their views
- group members committed to the task and willing to explore gaps in their knowledge
- students taking full responsibility of their learning
- students willing to become independent learners
- students seeing their effort to collect new information is not wasted and their contribution is useful to the group discussion
- students willing to evaluate their own strengths and weaknesses
- students willing to improve their self-directed learning approach
- students passionate about their learning.

→ KEY 8   TAKE RESPONSIBILITY FOR YOUR LEARNING

When people take responsibility of their own learning they:
- learn at a deeper level
- enjoy their learning
- become familiar with a range of learning strategies
- monitor their progress.

What does 'taking responsibility for your own learning' mean?
- Assume personal responsibility for planning learning activities.
- Think about mechanisms for carrying out these activities.
- Focus on the learning needs and the purpose of the learning activities.
- Have a clear vision of your learning needs.
- Capable of achieving your goals and assessing what you have accomplished.
- Able to identify key questions for the search.
- Able to identify the resources you will use.
- Able to analyse the information obtained and mentor your personal growth.
- Think about ways of enhancing your self-directed learning.

→ KEY 9 TURN LEARNING INTO AN ENJOYABLE EXPERIENCE

Turning self-directed learning into an enjoyable experience should be your paramount goal. Many students starting a PBL course feel that the new learning strategy is a burden and question its value. They may ask their course coordinators to use didactic teaching, provide them with learning issues or give them cues about what they need to learn. Other students find self-directed learning a great experience and enjoy their learning. The difference between the two groups is not because of a lack of knowledge about self-directed learning techniques; it is most likely caused by differences in perception. There is substantial evidence to show that when we reflect on what we enjoy most about our work we discover that our highest values are incorporated in it. This fuels our passion for our work and motivates us even further. Try it yourself. In your reflective journal, write down these statements and decide what you have enjoyed most.

> My favourite learning resource is …
> I feel my best when I am able to integrate information, see relationships between different disciplines and become aware of …
> My best time learning was …
> I can maximise my learning outcomes this year by …
> What I like most about my learning style this year is …
> My favourite learning experience is …
> My favourite multimedia CD-ROM is …
> The group I enjoy learning with is …
> I feel my best when I contribute effectively to my group discussion and …
> My long-term learning goals are …
> What I enjoyed most this week in PBL is …
> My greatest discovery learning moments were …

What are the positive experiences of self-directed learning?
Self-directed learners:
- feel they are in control
- decide on what they need to learn
- are passionate about their learning achievements
- are able to develop strategies for setting learning goals
- take an hypothesis-driven approach to their learning
- can debate different views
- are not compelled to use one particular resource
- are willing to research different aspects relating to a new concept
- are more able to apply information learnt in other situations
- can construct information from several resources
- are able to remember the knowledge they searched for several months ago
- are able to deal with uncertainty and provide justification for their views
- are able to remember these experiences after graduation.

➜ KEY 10 REVIEW WHAT YOU HAVE ACHIEVED

A review of what you have achieved enables you to:
- assess your learning performance
- assess your long-term growth and development
- improve your skills in areas of weakness
- foster your self-reinforcement and self-motivation.

Evaluate your self-directed learning.

Rank each skill/competency listed here using the ranking system below. Make sure that you have allocated your best estimate and that you are able to use the designated skill.

- Abilities and skills in designing an enquiry plan and asking good questions
- Ability to consider contributing and interfering factors
- Ability to identify learning needs, learning objectives and develop a learning plan
- Ability to select appropriate resources
- Ability to use resources, collect data, analyse findings and assess their application and significance
- Ability to construct information from a number of resources
- Ability to achieve learning goals
- Ability to assess performance and identify areas of weakness
- Ability to maintain growth and personal development to achieve learning goals.

1 = you believe that you do not possess this skill
2 = you believe you have low skills in this area
3 = you are not sure
4 = you have a medium ability in this area
5 = you have had experience and skills in this area for some time and you have demonstrated competency and efficiency

Modified from Knowles MS. Self-directed learning. New York: Association Press; 1975.

→ KEY 11 BECOME A GOAL-ORIENTED LEARNER

Goal–oriented learners:

- are active learners
- use learning to accomplish specific objectives
- possess a high self-motivating capacity
- focus on achievements
- use planning strategies to achieve their learning goals
- process information at a deeper level of understanding.

How can I become a goal-oriented learner?

- Be clear about your learning goals. Ensure they cover the skills and competencies you need for your learning stage.
- Turn your goals into a management plan.
- Always check that you have allocated appropriate time to achieve each of your daily goals.
- Continually evaluate what you are doing.
- Ensure that your daily and weekly learning goals contribute towards your long-term goals.

→ KEY 12 YOU HAVE UNLIMITED POTENTIAL

- Believe in your skills and abilities.
- Empower yourself with positive thoughts.
- Focus on your plan.
- Think about the final outcome.

Self-regulation

These actions reinforce your self-regulation:

- goal setting
- planning ahead
- implementing metacognitive and cognitive skills
- applying management strategies
- using learning resources effectively
- practising self-motivation
- developing organisational skills
- mastering time management
- using learning models effectively
- continually evaluating performance
- developing the habit of self-reinforcement
- monitoring growth and development.

CONCLUSIONS

Self-directed learning is an essential strategy for your growth and development. It is not just about searching for new information on your own or finding answers for your learning issues; it also means building a competency model for yourself to identify the skills and competencies you need. Use the keys outlined in this chapter to develop your self-directed strategy.

EVIDENCE-BASED LEARNING

Smoothing out transitions: how pedagogy influences medical students' achievement of self-regulated learning goals.

Many medical schools include in their goals for medical student education their graduates' ability to self-assess and self-regulate their education upon graduation and throughout their professional lives. This study explores links between medical students' use of self-regulated learning as it relates to motivation, autonomy, and control, and how these influenced their experiences in medical school. Subjects were medical students in two distinct medical school environments, 'Problem-based learning' and 'Traditional'. PBL students described a rough transition into medical school, but once they felt comfortable with the autonomy and control PBL gave them, they embraced the independence and responsibility. They found themselves motivated to learning for learning's sake, and able to channel their motivation into effective transitions from the classrooms into the clerkships. Traditional students had a rougher transition from the classrooms to the clerkships. In the first two years they relied on faculty to direct and control learning, and they channelled their motivation toward achieving the highest grade. In the clerkships, they found faculty expected them to be more independent and self-directed than they felt prepared to be, and they struggled to assume responsibility for their learning. Self-regulated learning can help smooth out the transitions through medical school by preparing first and second year students for expectations in the third and fourth years, which can then maximize learning in the clinical milieu, and prepare medical students for a lifetime of learning.

White CB. Adv Health Sci Educ Theory Prac 2006 Jun 10; [Epub ahead of print].
    Adapted with permission from the publisher.
For more information: http://www.springerlink.com/content/1573-1677/

FURTHER READING
BOOKS

Brockett RG, Hiemstra R. Self-direction in adult learning: perspectives in theory, research, and practice. New York: Routledge; 1991.
Candy PC. Self-direction for lifelong learning. San Francisco: Jossey–Bass; 1991.
Knowles M. Self-directed learning: a guide for learners and teachers. New York: Association Press, 1975.

ARTICLES AND RESEARCH PAPERS

Ainoda N, Onishi H, Yasuda Y. Definitions and goals of 'self-directed learning' in contemporary medical education literature. Ann Acad Med Singapore 2005; 34(8):515–519.
Blumberg P, Michael JA. Development of self-directed learning behaviours in a partially teacher-directed problem-based learning curriculum. Teach Learn Med 1992; 4:3–8.
Coles CR. Differences between conventional and problem-based curricula in their students' approaches to studying. Med Educ 1985; 19(4): 308–309.
Hmelo CE. Problem-based learning: effects on the early acquisition of cognitive skill in medicine. J Learn Sci 1998; 7(2):173–208.
Miser WF. Critical appraisal of the literature. J Am Board Fam Prac 1999; 12(4): 315–333.

CHAPTER 5

Learning issues

> Education is not how much you have committed to memory, or even how much you know. It's being able to differentiate between what you know and what you don't. **ANATOLE FRANCE**

INTRODUCTION

Problem-based learning (PBL) cases provide students with opportunities to discover areas in which their knowledge is deficient. These areas of deficiency are usually identified by students, not the tutor, and are called *learning issues*. Learning issues are those topics requiring further study outside the PBL tutorials. Identification of learning issues is a critical determinant of student success in studying and construction of appropriate knowledge, using self-directed learning skills. The process of identification is owned by the students and is central to PBL. The following factors affect the group's ability to identify appropriate learning issues:

- mechanisms used to explore difficult concepts such as asking good open-ended questions, using a medical dictionary and other resources, thinking laterally, weighing evidence when assessing hypotheses
- organisational skills of the scribe and group dynamics
- effective use of tutorial time
- discussion of progress in the case with no shortcuts or jumps
- contribution of each member to the discussion
- knowledge learnt from prior cases and lectures
- mechanisms used to resolve conflict
- time spent on editing the learning issues before leaving the tutorial
- facilitation skills of the tutor
- ability of the case writers to create a well-structured case reflecting the pre-set faculty-generated learning objectives. This factor is known as *problem effectiveness*.

In most PBL programs, the cases are written by a team with expertise in PBL, reviewed by the writing teams and evaluated by using questionnaires completed by students at the end of the case discussion. So the ability of the case writers to create a well-structured case is usually the factor with least impact on the identification process. In addition, all PBL programs use workshops to train tutors in standardised group facilitation, ensuring they have acquired the skills needed for this style of teaching. However, tutors can still vary a lot in their facilitating skills. Therefore the role of the group in identifying the appropriate learning issues is vital.

DEFINING LEARNING ISSUES

Learning issues of a PBL case must fulfil the following requirements:

- Learning issues are gaps of knowledge identified by students during the discussion of a PBL case.
- Learning issues are important concepts outlined during the case discussion (mainly in tutorial 1 of each case).
- The group feels that these issues are essential to their learning process and are relevant to the case discussed.
- Learning issues reflect integrated knowledge from different disciplines. A good example of a learning issue reflecting this is, 'Understand the relationship between the function and the structural features of the muscle cell'. This learning issue aims to integrate knowledge in the area of muscle physiology and histological structure and find the relationships included in this concept. It may be useful in discovering clinical applications and pathophysiological changes related to the case.

    In addition they should:
- be specific, clearly written as full sentences and highlight specific objectives
- build on what the group already knows
- highlight knowledge with relevance to the clinical practice
- highlight issues about which students have demonstrated misconceptions, incomplete understanding or disagreements
- be written on the whiteboard by the scribe and edited by the group before leaving the tutorial
- not be a long list of keywords.

TOP 10 PITFALLS

When students experience PBL for the first time, they can find tutorials very challenging because the process differs from what they are used to from their school days. Even though students have a wide range of learning strategies acquired during their schooling or from other life experiences, these strategies may not be sufficient for effective group discussion, identifying areas of deficiency in their learning and areas already known to them. As a result, groups can encounter a number of pitfalls in coming to grips with PBL. Here are the top 10 pitfalls.

PITFALL 1 SUPERFICIAL GROUP DISCUSSION

Group discussion may be superficial during the first few tutorials: students fail to address issues to the depth needed, thus compromising the quality of their learning and interfering with their ability to be specific about what they need to learn. The group may fail to: (1) ask good open-ended questions to broaden discussion; (2) use diagrams when needed to explain structures involved in their hypotheses; (3) explore contributing factors; or (4) list available evidence for their views. The tutor should help the group to explore these facilitating options.

PITFALL 2 IGNORING BASIC SCIENCES

This is a common problem in PBL tutorials. In most PBL cases the trigger describes patients presenting with three or four symptoms, so students may focus their hypotheses on commonly known illnesses and ignore basic sciences in their discussion. For example, students may identify the following problems from the trigger: (1) shortness of breath, (2) dizziness, and (3) loss of consciousness.

Their hypotheses for the shortness of breath might include asthma and heart problems. For the dizziness they might come up with low blood pressure, diabetes, ear trouble and side-effects of medications. For the loss of consciousness, they might come up with heart problems, epilepsy, fainting and low blood pressure.

Students usually find it difficult to add more hypotheses to their list. Asking questions such as: 'Do we have any other causes?' will not help students and may encourage guessing. If the group discussion is left as such, students will progress to the next task and will miss the opportunity to address basic sciences related to the case. This will impact on their ability to identify learning issues and they will miss out on including basic sciences in their search.

A good way to overcome this problem is to facilitate the discussion by asking good open-ended questions. If the tutor does not do this, here is the first of two key questions you might ask in such a situation: 'Normally we are not short of breath. What are the structures and functions we need so that we can breathe normally?'

With the help of a scribe, the group might start creating a list like this:

- Nose
- Larynx
- Trachea, bronchi
- Alveoli, lung tissue
- Pleural membranes (pleura)
- Pulmonary artery, aorta, other major arteries
- Heart
- Normal blood volume
- Central nervous system, nerves
- Brainstem.

The tutor might ask the group to provide detail about these structures. Using the resources available to them the group might add to 'Heart' the following: two atria, two ventricles, walls between the two atria and the two ventricles, valves (aortic, mitral, pulmonary, tricuspid) and muscles of the ventricles. The scribe could use a pen of a different colour to write the information.

To 'Normal blood volume' they might add: red blood cells, haemoglobin (because haemoglobin carries the oxygen).

The second open-ended question is: 'What could possibly go wrong and affect each of these structures causing shortness of breath?' Once again the group starts discussing this question and adding their new information. They might come up with the following:

- Nose ⇨ ? blocked nose, common cold
- Larynx ⇨ ? blocked by a tumour mass
- Trachea, bronchi ⇨ narrowed, constricted, decreased air entry (as in asthma)
- Alveoli, lung tissue ⇨ loss of alveoli, damaged or destroyed alveoli, thick walled (decreased gas exchange)
- Pleural membranes (pleura) ⇨ fluid or air in the pleural space
- Pulmonary artery, aorta, other major arteries ⇨ pulmonary artery blocked by a large blood thrombus (interfering with lung perfusion)
- Heart ⇨ failed muscles of ventricles, problems with valves (mitral, aortic, tricuspid or pulmonary), problem with the wall between the two ventricles

- Normal blood volume ⇨ loss of blood volume, anaemia (low haemoglobin, decreased oxygen-carrying capacity)
- Central nervous system, nerves ⇨ anxiety, panic
- Brainstem ⇨ problems affecting the respiratory centres in the brainstem (e.g. stroke, haemorrhage).

This approach can be used to expand discussion of the other two presenting symptoms, dizziness and loss of consciousness. Such discussion will help students to:
- understand the role of basic sciences in the case (mainly anatomy, physiology and pathophysiology)
- ask appropriate history questions to address each of their hypotheses
- refine their hypotheses as the case progresses and they receive new information from the medical history and clinical examination
- identify learning issues directly related to the objectives of the case.

PITFALL 3 FAILING TO USE RESOURCES DURING THE TUTORIAL

Each case adds new scientific terms to students' learning. They need to understand the meaning of the new terms and their significance in the context presented in the case. The use of the resources available to you in the PBL rooms such as medical dictionary, anatomy atlas, pharmacology resource book, textbooks and online resources are useful in understanding these terms and expanding the case discussion by using the new information learnt from these resources. New scientific terms that you might come across include blood pressure, ejection systolic murmur, fourth heart sound, palpitation, pulse rate, third heart sound.

The use of a medical dictionary, for example, might help you in expanding your discussion to the depth required. The PBL case scenario below outlines one such situation:

Tracy Ng, a 26-year-old primary school teacher is brought by ambulance to the emergency department of a local hospital. Tracy has fractured her left femur, tibia and fibula in a motor vehicle accident. She also has multiple lacerations on her body and has lost over 2 L of blood. Tracy has no history of medical problems. On examination, she is conscious but in pain. Her vital signs are as follows: blood pressure 80/60 mmHg (normal: 100/60–130/80 mmHg); pulse rate 105/min, regular (normal: 60–100/min); respiratory rate 24/min (normal 12–16/min); temperature 36.5°C (normal: 36.6–37.2°C). Cardiovascular and respiratory examinations are normal.

Let us assume that this case summary is presented to first-year medical students who have limited information about cardiovascular physiology. If the group uses one of the standard medical dictionaries to search for the new terms such as *blood pressure*, they might come up with the definition: 'Blood pressure or tension of blood within the systemic arteries, maintained by the contraction of the left ventricle, the resistance of the arterioles and capillaries, the elasticity of the arterial walls, as well as the viscosity and volume of the blood; expressed as relative to the ambient atmospheric pressure'. This definition was taken from p. 1423 of *Stedman's Medical Dictionary*. 26th edn. Philadelphia: Williams & Wilkins; 1995.

With the help of the scribe the group might list the factors affecting the normal blood pressure as per the definition: (1) force of contraction of the left ventricle,

(2) resistance of the arterioles and capillaries, (3) elasticity of the arterial walls, (4) blood viscosity, and (5) blood volume.

Then they might discuss which of these factors are most likely to have contributed to the patient's low blood pressure. Then they might move on and discuss other new terms and begin to see relationships between the new information and the case scenario.

PITFALL 4 FAILING TO ADDRESS EACH PROBLEM ON ITS OWN

Students may discuss all the problems together rather than discuss the hypotheses for each problem. They might construct one list of hypotheses for the three problems mentioned earlier: (1) shortness of breath, (2) dizziness, and (3) loss of consciousness. This might be because they cannot see any significant differences between dizziness and loss of consciousness or they are not aware about the time needed to complete the task discussed or because they have a tendency to take shortcuts and are more worried about the diagnosis than the discussion of the different components of the case.

Taking shortcuts will not help the group discussion and will make it very difficult to refine hypotheses and identify the most likely causes of the patient's problems. Such an approach will foster superficial learning and will give the impression to the students that the PBL case is not well written and does not address basic sciences or challenge students. You should always address each problem on its own and discuss hypotheses for each problem. If the same hypothesis is repeated under two or three problems, this will be useful when you start ranking your hypotheses and identifying the body system responsible for the patient's problems.

PITFALL 5 FOCUSING ON UNRELATED OR PERIPHERAL ISSUES

Some students see learning as isolated pieces of factual knowledge that they need to memorise for examinations. They fail to link the knowledge learnt, see the relationships between different concepts and apply the knowledge they have learnt from other situations.

Other students may focus on peripheral issues and the fine details and not maintain a balance in their discussion between the big picture and the fine details. For example, students may spend 20–30 minutes discussing the Na^+, K^+–ATPase transporter and arguing whether Na^+ is pumped out of the cell or into the cell, what changes will happen to the Na^+ and K^+ as a result, whether 2 or 3 Na^+ ions are used and other similar details. These details are important to your learning but spending 20 minutes on them in a PBL tutorial is not useful. Using a CD-ROM or searching a physiology textbook or an educational website outside the PBL tutorial will provide you with all you need to know about this transporter. The discussion in PBL should be focused on key principles related to this area, for example: (1) What are the key physiological principles behind the location and function of the active transporters? (2) Why do we need primary and secondary transporters in these cells? and (3) What are the different transporters responsible for moving substances across the cell membrane?

PITFALL 6 NOT USING TUTORIAL TIME EFFECTIVELY

One of the keys for successful PBL discussion is using tutorial time effectively. Students need to develop this skill and learn how to spend enough time on the different aspects of the case. Your tutor will be guiding the group in the first two or three tutorials but they eventually will leave this responsibility to the group and you should always raise the question when you start a new task, 'How much time should we spend discussing this issue?' Your tutor might suggest the time needed: one of the students in the group could be the timekeeper and warn the group if they exceed the allotted time.

PITFALL 7 FAILING TO USE A SCRIBE AT ALL
OR EFFECTIVELY

Some groups may discuss the case without a scribe and thus not record the issues raised during the discussion. The problems with this approach include:
*   failure to follow up what has already been discussed
*   members repeat what has already been said
*   difficulty in using the new information obtained from the history and clinical examination to rank and prioritise hypotheses
*   failure to use the tutorial time effectively. The group may lose focus; some members may dominate the discussion
*   contribution of members in the group gradually decreases; some may lose interest
*   because the group is not drawing diagrams or constructing flow charts or tables to compare and summarise issues raised, understanding will decrease. Members will find it difficult to discuss issues to the depth needed.

For all these reasons it is important to have a scribe in PBL tutorials. The role of a scribe is vital to the success of tutorials and every student in the group should be encouraged to undertake this role on a regular basis.

PITFALL 8 FAILING TO REASSESS KNOWLEDGE AND
ACCUMULATED EVIDENCE

There is a tendency in some groups to ignore issues discussed and fail to build on the information created as the case progresses. A good example is: when asked to identify history questions they would ask the patient, students ignore the hypotheses they have discussed and instead identify questions unrelated to their earlier discussion. A better approach is to look at each of your hypotheses and think about questions that would either confirm or exclude each hypothesis.

Another example is the failure of the group to rank their hypotheses and list them under two main headings, 'Most likely causes' and 'Least likely causes'. This is usually because they ignore the key information provided to them in the medical history and clinical examination. The lesson here is: when ranking your hypotheses, you need to reassess key information and cues provided in the history and examination and evaluate their significance before making any decisions.

PITFALL 9 FAILING TO TAKE ON ROLES

Some groups fail to endorse ground rules, or the rules they do have are not related to group organisational and management issues. For example, (1) Every member should contribute to the discussion; (2) Every member should take on roles that rotate among members. These rules should be turned into an action plan and members can, for example, agree with their tutor to use the attendance sheet for the fair allocation of roles.

PITFALL 10 FAILING TO RECOGNISE NEW ASPECTS OF THE CASE

This is typically seen in students who have covered topics in other courses they have completed that are similar to those being presented in the PBL case. For example, a PBL case covers the following issues: excessive loss of sweat, exposure to high environmental temperature, electrolyte imbalance and physiological mechanisms of body homeostasis. Students in the PBL tutorial may have studied similar issues in the undergraduate biomedical science course they completed before being accepted into the medical course. When encountering a case covering these contents in the medical course students may say, 'Oh yeah, I know everything about this area'. In other words, they assume they have enough knowledge and do not need to study it again in the medical course. They might say to themselves, 'There is nothing new to me here. It is great that I know all these issues'. Therefore, little or no attention is paid to revisiting these concepts. The problems created by such an attitude include:

- failure to realise that there are new issues you need to study. You may have learnt similar concepts in a science course but the focus here is different
- failure to acknowledge the need to learn these concepts to the depth required by the medical course. In a PBL medical course you may need to learn: (1) how to apply knowledge learnt to real-life situations, (2) how to use supportive evidence, (3) how to integrate information across disciplines, (4) how to use basic sciences to explain the patient's signs and symptoms, (5) what type of investigations you need to order, (6) what your management goals should be and how to construct a management plan, and (7) the impact of these problems on the patient
- failure to adjust your learning style to the needs of the PBL course.

WHAT TO AVOID IN LEARNING ISSUES

Although there is no specific way to construct your learning issues and each group has its own ways of creating them, there are a number of things you should avoid:

- broad, non-specific and unrealistic learning issues such as anatomy and physiology of the cardiovascular system
- learning issues not related directly to the case discussed
- fragmented, discipline-based learning issues
- statements that focus on theory and ignore clinical application
- a long list of keywords or scientific terms mentioned in the case
- learning issues that do not address cognitive skills and understanding, such as the evidence you have, structural functional relationships and pathogenesis and mechanisms
- learning issues that do not raise the key educational principles behind the case

- learning issues that focus on one aspect of the case
- learning issues that lack purpose.

Learning issues are constructed by the group and they are the outcome of your group discussion. Learning how to avoid pitfalls is vital and the group should evaluate their performance at the end of each case. The following keys will help you and your group construct useful learning issues that improve your self-directed learning.

KEYS FOR SUCCESSFUL IDENTIFICATION OF LEARNING ISSUES

If we would have new knowledge, we must get a whole world of new questions.

SUSANNE K. LANGER

The time for releasing the pre-set faculty-generated learning objectives varies between universities. For example, some universities release the learning objectives at the beginning of the unit or semester. This is usually in a case-based curriculum. In other universities, learning objectives are released after students complete the tutorial 1 discussion and have identified their learning issues. Others release the learning objectives at the end of each case, at the end of the unit, the semester or approximately 2–3 weeks before the summative examination. Others do not release the pre-set faculty-generated learning objectives at all. It has been reported that students most frequently use the faculty-generated objectives as a checklist at the end of the case to ensure they have covered all the relevant topics. When the students find they have not covered an objective, they learn this material independently or make it a group learning issue to be addressed briefly the week after.

The following keys for successful identification of learning issues will be of particular use to students not receiving the pre-set faculty-generated learning objectives before discussing the case.

→ KEY 1 DEBATE/NEGOTIATE WITH YOUR GROUP

Your group might start identifying the learning issues at an early stage of discussion of the case, for example, during the discussion of the trigger or history sections. As the case progresses, you might need to amend or change your learning issues. For instance, the patient as per the trigger has upper abdominal pain. The group identifies 'peptic ulcer' as one of their learning issues. The group might state the learning issue for this as 'Do we understand the pathogenesis of pain in peptic ulcer?' As the case progresses, the group notices that the patient has had a history of shortness of breath and high blood pressure and there are signs suggestive of myocardial infarction. The group needs to negotiate these changes. They might omit the learning issue 'Do we understand the pathogenesis of pain in peptic ulcer?' and replace it with two new learning issues 'Do we understand the pathogenesis and pathology of myocardial infarction?' and 'What is the pathogenesis of pain in acute myocardial infarction/ ischaemia?' However, all group members may not agree on these changes. It is essential to spend time debating, negotiating (collaborating) about whether or not each item should be added to the list of learning issues.

Good negotiation strategies require:
- effective communication
- listening to other members in the group

- justification of your views
- focusing on issues, not people
- dealing with obstacles
- collaboration in the decision-making process
- reaching an agreement.

➜ KEY 2 STRUCTURE LEARNING ISSUES AS COMPLETE SENTENCES

The learning issues need to be written in dot points as complete sentences. They can be in question format. They should not be in the form of a list of keywords or brief statements. We need to write learning issues in full to:

- highlight key points to be researched
- ensure integration across disciplines
- sharpen the research objectives
- make learning issues meaningful
- link basic sciences and clinical issues
- be specific about what is needed from each member.

➜ KEY 3 LINK BASIC AND CLINICAL SCIENCES

The whole aim of the learning issues and your search is not just learning about theory and basic medical sciences but to explore related clinical knowledge. Why is it important to link basic and clinical sciences in your learning issues?

- One of the aims of PBL cases is to prepare students for clinical years.
- Explaining the scientific basis behind a patient's presenting symptoms and clinical signs will help you understand the pathophysiological and pathological changes, possible preventive measures and the basis of your management plan.
- You will understand the significance of knowledge learnt from basic sciences such as anatomy, biochemistry, histology, microbiology, pharmacology, pathology and physiology.
- You will be more able to retain the information learnt in your long-term memory.
- You will be more able to identify investigations needed and interpret the laboratory and radiological changes.

  Examples of learning issues linking basic and clinical sciences:

- What caused his low blood calcium, high parathyroid hormone and high phosphate levels? What are the mechanisms underlying these changes? Could these changes explain his bone pains? How?
- What are the mechanisms by which water is absorbed from the large and small intestine? What are the mechanisms by which diarrhoea occurs? Is his diarrhoea due to a functional or pathological change? What evidence do I have so far? What type of investigations could help? How?
- What are the possible causes for her palpitation, pallor and progressive tiredness? How can I explain her low haemoglobin? How are red blood cells formed in the body? What other investigations do I need to order? How can these investigations help?

→ KEY 4 CONSIDER PSYCHOSOCIAL, MORAL AND ETHICAL ISSUES

Why do you study psychosocial, moral and ethical issues?

- Many of the problems encountered in our communities are related to psychosocial, ethical and moral issues.
- Skills, attitudes and competencies in these areas are required for medical and healthcare practice.
- Medical ethics and law constitutes one of the core components of the medical and healthcare curricula.
- You are required to adhere to the beliefs and values of the profession.
- In real-life situations, you cannot separate basic and clinical science knowledge from ethical and psychosocial competencies.

There are a number of factors that affect our decision making in moral and ethical problems. These factors can be summarised as:

- our own beliefs and cultural beliefs
- common sense
- science knowledge
- current laws
- professional codes and guidelines
- theories and research in the area.

During the course you will learn: (1) what questions these problems raise, (2) how to approach these challenges, (3) what resources are available to you about such situations and how to assess these resources, (4) what options are available, (5) what type of support is available, and (6) what strategies you can use in such situations.

→ KEY 5 BE SPECIFIC AND HIGHLIGHT INTEGRATION

Integrating knowledge in the learning issues is not easy to do. It might take your group some time to clearly specify what you need to learn and how to present your learning issues in an integrated and meaningful manner.

Examples of integration in learning issues:

- structural functional relationships and clinical implications. For example, 'How do liver cells handle bilirubin?' 'How could this explain the development of his jaundice?'
- normal physiological mechanisms and the development of pathophysiological changes. For example, 'What are the mechanisms controlling normal blood pressure? How can we explain her low blood pressure and rapid pulse rate after the motor vehicle accident?'
- explaining the mechanisms by which drugs work by using knowledge learnt from physiology. For example, 'How does the kidney handle water?' 'What are the mechanisms by which frusemide works?'
- using the pathogenesis of the disease to develop a management plan. For example, 'What are the mechanisms by which pulmonary oedema develops?' 'How could the management actions reverse these changes?'
- differences between normal structure and pathological changes. For example, 'What is the normal lining of the colon?' 'How can we explain the cellular

changes demonstrated in the biopsy?'
- role of biochemical changes in the pathogenesis of a disease. For example, 'What are the changes caused by alcohol?' 'Could these changes explain the fluid in his abdomen (ascites)?' 'How?'
- microbiological knowledge, clinical picture and disease development. For example, 'How can we explain his fever, lethargy, loss of appetite and the local redness/pain in his left ankle?'

→ KEY 6 AMEND, EDIT AND FINALISE

The aims in amending, editing and finalising learning issues are to:
- strengthen the learning issue items and their objectives
- avoid repetition and redundant items
- clarify items and make them more specific
- omit unrelated items or place them at the end of the list
- introduce integration and add clinical significance to some items
- link related items
- identify the most important four or five learning issues.

APPROACHES FOR COLLECTION OF INFORMATION

In my work in two universities, a number of students came to see me because they wanted to improve their performance in the summative examinations and enhance their contribution to the PBL discussion. Their questions were focused on: 'How should we prepare our learning issues?' 'How can we be effective in our approach and able to master the self-directed learning component?' Some of these students were troubled with the time they spent reading their medical textbooks and other resources. Their problems were: 'Why, despite our effort and hard work, do we find it difficult to contribute to the group discussion? At times we feel we did not read or prepare enough and all our effort is wasted. We do not feel that we are making any progress.'

I looked at samples of their preparation for the PBL cases and asked them to describe what they do as they prepare their learning issues. I listened to them. Then I asked them to use the textbooks in my room and show me their approach as they searched for information and recorded their findings. It was clear that their main problems were related to their approach and the way they used resources in their preparation. In the following section I deal with the questions commonly asked by students about preparation of learning issues.

HOW DO I PREPARE MY LEARNING ISSUES?

- Start by reviewing the learning issues identified by your group.
- Read the PBL case you have discussed in tutorial 1 and review the notes taken in the tutorial.
- Before you start your search, spend some time on: (1) asking key questions that will help you refine your hypotheses if the group has ended tutorial 1 with two or three hypotheses and is not sure of a final one, (2) adding sub-questions that may offer new dimensions to your understanding of each learning issue, and (3) turning your learning issues into learning objectives.

- Look at the list of resources; if your faculty provides you with a list use it in organising your search.
- Think about these questions, and write down your answers: (1) Which resource should I start using? (2) What keywords should I use in my search? (3) What type of information am I looking at? and (4) What are the other resources I may use?
- Search the textbook index using the keywords you have identified. Your keywords should reflect the learning issues. Also examine the contents page for extra information. Record the page numbers and related sub-entries you have identified.
- Look at your lecture notes and review information related to the learning items you are searching.
- Some cases address issues related to anatomy, biochemistry, pathology and physiology. You should be able to identify these aspects of your learning issues.
- Always ask yourself, 'Are there any psychosocial, ethical or moral issues raised in the case?' Apply the strategies discussed earlier: (1) What questions do these ethical/psychosocial issues raise? (2) What approach should I take? (3) What are the resources available to me about such challenges and how do I use these resources? (4) What are the available options? (5) What type of support is available? and (6) What strategies would I use in dealing with such a situation?

HOW DO I SEARCH IN RESOURCES?

There is a wide range of resources you can use in searching for your learning issues. As mentioned earlier, textbooks and educational websites may be your primary resource. However, you will notice that textbooks may have limitations:

- Most textbooks are discipline-based but in a PBL curriculum you need to integrate issues across disciplines.
- Textbooks present information linearly, one piece at a time, but you need to understand how different pieces fit together.
- Many textbooks focus on theory and ignore clinical applications of the topics they present but you need to use information learnt and apply it to specific cases.
- Textbooks cannot present the big picture because of their specialisation and each text focuses on only one aspect of what you need.
- Many textbooks have gaps; they may not answer all your questions.

I mention these limitations so you don't think that it is your fault if you have difficulty reading a textbook. Everyone does. What is more important here is how to use textbooks effectively, particularly when your goal is not to read and memorise the text provided in a textbook.

Your primary goals are to:
- search for useful information
- find answers to your learning issues
- understand new concepts and principles
- learn from a number of resources and construct your own information
- provide justification for your views
- weigh the evidence for and against different hypotheses
- apply knowledge learnt to new problems.

With these aims in mind, your approach to using learning resources will be different from that used in a traditional course. Table 5.1 summarises the main differences.

TABLE 5.1 Comparison of textbook use in traditional and PBL curricula

Traditional curriculum	PBL curriculum
Students are aware of the topics discussed in the lectures and have no learning issues.	Students are not sure of the final hypotheses and have a list of learning issues.
Students read discipline-based textbooks to learn more about issues covered in the lectures.	Students search several resources covering a number of disciplines to find answers for their learning issues.
Students have few prior questions.	Students have thought of a number of questions from their learning issues and planned their search.
Students follow the sequence of information as outlined by the author.	Most of the time students are trying to find answers to their questions. They may scan the text, tables and diagrams provided in the order they find most useful.
Students learn for memorisation of factual knowledge.	Students learn for understanding key concepts, providing justification, reasoning and applying knowledge to the case.
Students use the contents page of each textbook to find the chapter title.	Students search the textbook index using keywords.
Students aim to summarise the pages they read.	Students aim to integrate information learnt and construct flow charts and tables to suit their learning needs.
Students are less likely to be challenged by new questions.	The new information learnt from several resources and the case raises new questions for the learner and improves their search.
There is no opportunity for discussing information learnt with other students.	The new information learnt will be discussed with other members in tutorial 2.

Let's say you're having trouble understanding the cardiac cycle. What to do? You could struggle with it for hours, or you could seek out another resource for information. Do not limit your search to one resource. Check educational websites and other useful resources (see Appendices A and B). Check journal articles, review papers, educational CD-ROMs, educational videos, lecture notes and any resources provided—anything that helps you understand the learning issues and the case. Using other textbooks in the same discipline is usually of great value. Remember, each author approaches a subject from a different point of view, explains it differently, emphasises different aspects and provides different diagrams, tables and explanations.

The advantages of using multiple resources in self-directed learning are to:
- improve your reasoning capabilities by providing you with additional information
- enhance your understanding of different concepts and processes
- develop your thinking and leave you with more than one point of view
- provide you with more examples and clinical applications for the topics you are searching
- throw new light on concepts you misunderstood.

LEARNING ISSUES AND CONSTRUCTION OF INFORMATION

According to the traditional theory of learning, the learner's mind contains images that represent copies or pictures of what the teacher presented. This does not guarantee deep learning or the ability of the learner to debate, justify or apply information learnt. Traditional theory has shaped the way classrooms are designed and courses are run: students sit facing the teacher who is the sole source of knowledge.

With the *constructive theory of learning*, the learner does not mirror and repeat what they are told or what they read. According to this theory, learners search for meaning, collect information from a wide range of resources, comprehend what they have learnt, test the new knowledge and try to find relationships, organise the information learnt and construct this knowledge in their mind. This theory constitutes part of the teaching philosophy of the PBL curriculum. It is particularly useful when students discuss their learning issues in tutorial 2. Students should not underestimate the value of this session by, for instance, spending time drawing a diagram they copied from a textbook. Instead, they should work together to construct the knowledge they came up with.

A scribe who records this information will facilitate the process and help the group achieve their goals. The use of mechanisms in PBL can offer students the opportunity to construct their own mechanisms at the end of tutorial 2. Students will then be able to: (1) integrate knowledge needed for the construction of their mechanism from related disciplines such as biochemistry, microbiology, molecular biology, pathology, pharmacology, physiology; (2) include contributing factors or risk factors mentioned in the case scenario into their mechanism; (3) build their mechanism in a way that shows a logical flow of information with no shortcuts; (4) demonstrate understanding of the sequence of events (pathogenesis) at body system, organ, cellular and molecular levels; (5) show how their knowledge in other disciplines is addressed as they link it to their mechanism, to a drug action, side-effects or drug interaction; and (6) address the final target of their mechanism. (Construction and use of mechanisms and pathogenesis flow charts are covered in Ch 6.)

WHAT TO DO IF YOUR GROUP GENERATES NO FINAL HYPOTHESIS

Many times the group will not be able to reach a final hypothesis and will leave the PBL room with two or three hypotheses for the patient's problems.

Preparing your learning issues for such cases may be challenging for you because you need to find the most likely hypothesis then focus your learning issues on it. You will also need to provide supportive evidence for your views and why the other hypotheses are less likely. Preparing learning issues for such cases will require more work from you. However, the approach to a challenge like this can vary and there is no one answer. Some students will try to find a clue from the list of resources provided at the end of tutorial 1 or from the lectures they attended that week. But sometimes you cannot find a clue and you have to work it out on your own. This experience will strengthen your self-directed learning and will add new dimensions to your work.

The following example provides you with a similar situation. The discussion after the case should provide you with key principles for how to deal with such situations.

Mr Sam Mansour, a 65-year-old pensioner, comes in with his son to see his GP because of progressive shortness of breath over the last 6–8 months, recent dizziness and loss of consciousness twice over the last 10 days. On further questioning, he says, 'I noticed that I become short of breath when I walk my grandson to school, about 10 minutes walk from our house or when I do work at home. This has been getting progressively worse'. He at times feels dizzy and has lost consciousness twice, the most recent being yesterday. His son says that his father lost consciousness for a few minutes. Mr Mansour recalls no warnings such as dizziness, chest pain or sweating. But he occasionally has palpitations.

He occasionally drinks and he used to smoke 20 cigarettes per day but he stopped about 15 years ago. He has a history of pneumothorax when he was 18 years old. His father died of a heart attack at the age of 68.

On examination: his pulse is 70/min and of poor volume, his blood pressure is 105/85 mmHg on sitting and 100/85 on standing, his respiratory rate is 20/min and he is afebrile.

Cardiovascular examination reveals: normal jugular venous pressure; his apex beat in the 5th left intercostal space is inside the midclavicular line; his first heart sound is normal but the second heart sound is soft. A fourth heart sound and an ejection systolic murmur are heard over the pericardium. The murmur is heard over the two carotid arteries. No other abnormalities are found.

Students were unable to identify a final hypothesis. Their most likely hypotheses were: (1) pulmonary valve disease, (2) aortic stenosis, (3) aortic regurgitation, (4) left-sided heart failure, and (5) mitral valve stenosis.

The group identified the following learning issues:

- What is the anatomy of the heart and the circulation of blood in the heart and lungs?
- Do we understand the exchange of gases in lungs?
- The normal (S_1 and S_2) and abnormal heart sounds (S_3 and S_4): what causes them and their significance.
- What changes occur during systole and diastole?
- How can we explain his problems—shortness of breath, dizziness and loss of consciousness—and the pathogenesis of his problems?
- What is the supportive evidence for the final hypothesis?

Now, going to the original question, what would you do to identify the final hypothesis for Mr Mansour's presentation? Table 5.2 summarises six key questions that you might use to refine your hypothesis. Notice the logical flow of the key questions and the relationships between the main and learning questions. During this process you might think about new questions similar to those I have listed. You could also solve this challenge by constructing a table similar to that of Table 5.3 (see later).

TABLE 5.2 Key questions and their answers

Key questions	Possible discussion questions	Answers and new learning questions
Question 1	Is this a respiratory or a cardiovascular problem?	*Answer*: A cardiovascular problem *Evidence*: History of palpitation Low pulse pressure (105–85 = 20 mmHg) (normally it is about 40 mmHg) Pulse is of poor volume Cardiac auscultation: soft S_2, S_4 is heard, ejection systolic murmur is heard over the pericardium and over the two carotids *Learning question*: What is the structure and function of the normal heart?
Question 2	If this a heart problem, is this a right- or left-sided problem?	*Answer*: A left-sided heart problem *Evidence*: Left-sided heart problem is suggested by: — Poor pulse volume — Low pulse pressure — Murmur is heard on the pericardium and the two carotids (carotid arteries originate from the arch of the aorta) *Learning questions*: What is against a right-sided heart problem? What will the clinical picture be if it is a right-sided heart problem?
Question 3	On the left side, we mentioned a number of structures. Which one could be responsible? Mitral valve Aortic valve Left ventricular muscle Interventricular septum	*Answer*: The likely site of the problem is the aortic valve *Evidence*: The ejection systolic murmur is heard over the pericardium and over the two carotids This is the same murmur radiated from the aortic valve to the aortic arch to both carotids in the neck Together with poor pulse volume and low pulse pressure *Learning questions*: What is the normal structure of the aortic valve? What is against a mitral valve problem? What are the normal heart sounds? What is the mechanism by which heart sounds occur? What are the main differences between S_3 and S_4? What are the main physiological changes occurring during systole and diastole? What will the clinical picture be if the patient has a problem with left ventricular muscle?

continued

TABLE 5.2 Key questions and their answers *continued*

Key questions	Possible discussion questions	Answers and new learning questions
Question 4	What are the pathological changes?	*Answer*: Aortic valve stenosis *Evidence*: Usually the murmur of aortic stenosis is harsh and is maximal over the aortic area and extends into the carotid arteries Other causes of midsystolic murmur are: — Pulmonary stenosis — Hypertrophic cardiomyopathy — Pulmonary flow murmur of atrial septal defect While pansystolic murmur is heard in: — Mitral incompetence — Tricuspid incompetence — Ventricular septal defect *Learning questions*: What are the causes of aortic valve stenosis? What is the impact of these changes on the left ventricle function? What will be the clinical picture if the patient has aortic valve regurgitation?
Question 5	What are the pathophysiological changes?	*Answer*: Pathophysiological changes are summarised in a flow diagram See Figure 5.1 *Learning questions*: How could the aortic valvular changes explain his dizziness, shortness of breath and loss of consciousness? How can we explain the occurrence of his symptoms in hot weather? With exercise, and when is he emotionally affected?
Question 6	What are the investigations needed for this patient?	*Answer*: *Investigations*: — Full blood examination: to exclude anaemia — 12-lead ECG: left ventricular hypertrophy, down sloping of ST segments and T inversion (strain pattern) — Doppler and echocardiography: allows calculation of the systolic gradient across the aortic valve. To assess that other valves are not affected, measure valve area — CT and MRI scans: to assess the degree of valve calcification and stenosis (not usually needed) — Cardiac catheterisation: to assess the coronary arteries before the surgery *Learning questions*: How can these investigations help? What are the changes expected to be found in each of these investigations? What are the management goals?

TABLE 5.2 Key questions and their answers *continued*

Key questions	Possible discussion questions	Answers and new learning questions
New questions/comments: Are there any psychosocial, ethical or moral issues here? How can I apply what I learnt from this case in other cardiac problems?		

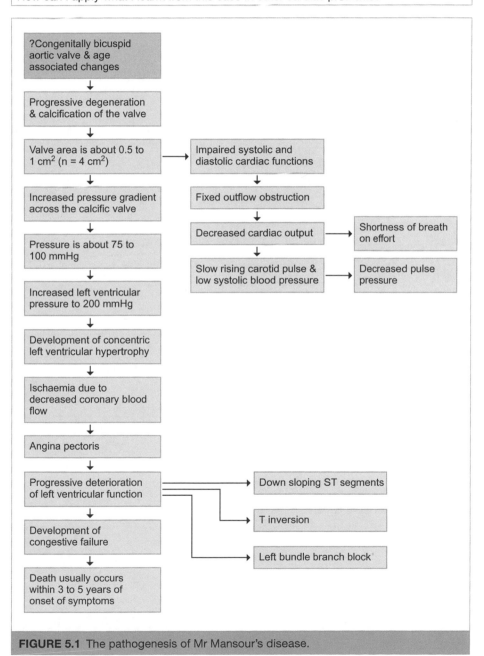

FIGURE 5.1 The pathogenesis of Mr Mansour's disease.

KEYS FOR SUCCESSFUL PREPARATION OF LEARNING ISSUES

> Employ your time in improving yourself by other men's writings, so that you shall gain easily what others have laboured hard for. SOCRATES

The keys in this section are all in the form of questions you need to ask yourself.

→ KEY 1 WHAT IS YOUR PURPOSE?

When you learn with a purpose you are:
- more able to achieve your goals in the time allocated for the task
- passionate about your learning
- focused and clear about what you need to do
- creative and empowered in the way you learn
- enjoy what you are doing
- willing to improve your performance
- giving learning a priority
- planning and designing for the goals you would like to achieve
- investing in your skills and building up your competencies
- committed to your work.

→ KEY 2 WHAT DID YOU LEARN IN TUTORIAL 1?

Go through the contents of the case scenario and review the notes taken during tutorial 1.

Think about these questions:
- What are the key principles raised in this case?
- What are the main points we discussed in tutorial 1?
- What does this case add to what I already know from previous cases?
- Why did we study this case?
- What are the new issues raised in this case?

If your group did not come up with a final hypothesis and you ended with two or three most likely causes, try to find clues in the case that can help you in the process.

Think about these questions:
- How long did the patient have these symptoms? Is this an acute or chronic problem?
- Were the patient's symptoms due to physiological or pathological changes? What evidence do I have to support my views?
- What is the significance of each of his symptoms?
- What exactly was his present illness? Are there any contributing factors to the patient's illness?
- What was significant in the medical history?
- Was the patient on any medication? Is there any drug interaction?
- Was the illness related to any family history? Is there any genetic basis for the disease?
- Was the patient's illness related to environmental or occupational reasons or exposure to any toxins?

- What was the social history of the patient?
- Is there any other information I need to know?

Review your notes and what your group has agreed on as hypotheses. Do you want to make any changes? Read the clinical history and answer the questions given to you.

Think about these questions:

- Are there any difficult terms I need to look up?
- What are the clinical examination findings? What is the significance of the changes found?
- Which body system is responsible for the patient's symptoms?

If you still find it difficult to refine your hypotheses and identify the most likely hypothesis, I recommend that you weigh the evidence for and against each hypothesis you have. Let's assume that the most likely hypotheses are: (1) pulmonary valve disease, (2) aortic stenosis, (3) aortic regurgitation, (4) left-sided heart failure, and (5) mitral valve stenosis.

Construct a table and use it as a tool in your assessment.

TABLE 5.3 A blueprint to weigh the evidence for and against each hypothesis

Evidence	Hypothesis 1 (pulmonary valve disease)	Hypothesis 2 (aortic stenosis)	Hypothesis 3 (aortic regurgitation)	Hypothesis 4 (left-sided heart failure)	Hypothesis 5 (mitral valve stenosis)
For:					
1. History					
2. Clinical examination findings					
Against:					
1. History					
2. Clinical examination findings					
Ranking					

In the table write in dot-point form the evidence from the medical history and clinical examination for and against each hypothesis.

When you complete the table look at the accumulated evidence and rank your hypotheses accordingly. Note: you might not be able to complete the whole table at this stage and reach a final conclusion.

→ KEY 3 WHAT IS THE BIG PICTURE?

- If you want to summarise the key principles you learnt in tutorial 1, what would you say?
- What is the big picture in this case?
- How does this case link with what you have already learnt from previous cases?

Refining your hypotheses will allow you to focus your thinking and identify new questions for your learning, but you are not quite ready to begin a close inspection of your textbooks and other resources. To understand something you need to see the whole concept first, then examine the fine details. Your aim is to prepare yourself for what you need to do: to look at the broad outline of the case and how this case links with what you already know.

→ KEY 4 WHICH CONCEPTS DO YOU NOT KNOW?

- What are the learning issues identified by your group?
- How would you turn the learning issues into learning objectives?
- Are there any sub-questions or new questions you need to add to the list?
- How will you start your search? What are the main keywords for your search?

→ KEY 5 WHICH KEY RESOURCES WILL YOU USE?

Many students start by searching textbooks, others start with educational websites such as eMedicine (www.emedicine.com), MedicineNet (www.medicinenet.com), MedicineOnline (www.medicineonline.com) or other online research resources. See Appendix A for a full list of these resources.

There is no rule about which book you should start with but it makes sense to start with a textbook in medicine if the PBL case you are studying addresses adult problems and a textbook in paediatrics if the case addresses children's problems. These resources may help you to:

- identify and learn more about the two or three hypotheses identified by your group as 'most likely hypotheses'
- ask yourself key questions that may help refine your hypotheses if your group did not come up with a final hypothesis
- understand the basic anatomy, physiology, pathology, biochemistry, microbiology, pharmacology related to the case
- think about the investigations you may need to order, how these investigations could help you and what changes you would expect.

Then you might search other textbooks covering basic sciences related to the final hypothesis. This search may provide you with an in-depth understanding of the case.

Most universities using PBL do not provide students with a list of recommended resources but if your university has recommended resources, it is preferable to start with those. Not all students use the recommended resources, preferring to use alternative material that suits their learning needs. Most students use about 7 to 20 resources.

→ KEY 6 HOW CAN YOU USE SELF-DIRECTED LEARNING TIME EFFECTIVELY?

With good time management skills you are:

- able to accomplish more with less stress
- able to maintain a balance between study, personal, family and work
- able to deal with unexpected situations
- aware of your priorities and focused on your achievements
- able to overcome obstacles that may be responsible for your *procrastination* (putting off the things you should be doing)

- not waiting for the right mood or the right time to do the work
- developing a habit that is essential for life-long success.

Procrastination is the result of many causes, the main ones being lack of planning, organisation and time management. Other causes can include:

- no clear goals/objectives
- too busy with many tasks
- underestimating time needed to complete a task
- no sense of ownership for what you are doing
- lack of motivation
- fear of failure.

Think about these questions:

- Do you feel that you are in control?
- Do you organise your time and plan what you want to do?
- How do you organise your time to get the best from self-directed learning?
- How many hours do you plan to spend on your search?
- What are your priorities for this week?
- Do you keep a reflective journal to record what you plan to do?
- What exactly do you record?
- Have you noticed any progress in your performance?
- Is there anything you need to change?

→ KEY 7 WHAT ARE THE KEY CONCEPTS?

Searching resources should be an active process in which you should aim to:

- understand basic principles about the topics you are searching
- consolidate main principles into meaningful statements
- analyse information learnt and measure differences in your findings
- interpret findings and identify contributing factors for the problems
- assess the process and predict changes that may occur
- identify deficiencies in your resources and areas that need further work
- identify possible underlying mechanisms and pathophysiological changes
- understand the clinical application of knowledge learnt and its potential use in solving problems.

Think about these questions:

- What does this information mean to you?
- Does this information answer your questions? What is missing?
- Does it justify your views? What evidence do you have so far?
- What else do you need to know?
- Are you able to summarise the information you have learnt from these resources?
- How can this information be applied to clinical situations?
- How can this information be used to address your learning issues?

→ KEY 8 HOW DO YOU CONSTRUCT THE NEW INFORMATION?

There is a strong body of evidence that we understand complex ideas and modes of inquiry when we learn by doing and actively engage our minds. Thus, construction and organisation of information learnt from several resources is another skill you need to develop. This process can include:

- constructing tables for comparing issues that share common ground
- building mechanisms and flow charts
- synthesising concept maps
- designing an analogy model to illustrate difficult concepts
- creating diagrams to illustrate structural and functional relationships, pathological changes, complex sequences of events and relationships
- constructing three-dimensional models to explain difficult concepts and procedures
- using colours to outline surface anatomy
- applying information learnt to new problems
- using information learnt to answer short-answer questions, PBL-style questions or objective structured clinical examination (OSCE) questions.

The knowledge you created should not be copied from one particular resource; rather, it should reflect your own understanding, interpretation, accumulated experiences and use of the new knowledge. Because the new tables, figures, mechanisms and so on are your own creation, they are retained in your long-term memory and you will be able to use the information learnt in other situations.

→ KEY 9 HOW DO YOU CONNECT NEW INFORMATION WITH WHAT YOU ALREADY KNOW?

- How does the case scenario help you to hook the new information?
- What links the new information learnt?
- How does the new information relate to what you already know?
- How do the issues raised in this case relate to previous PBL cases?
- How would you summarise the relationship between the new knowledge in the current case and previous cases?

Here are examples of relationships and how the new information links with what was learnt from previous cases.

- In week 3, we had a case on prolonged starvation and metabolic changes in the body during starvation; an interesting issue in the case was the changes in the patient's laboratory tests including blood urea.
- In week 5, we had the case of a patient brought by ambulance to the emergency department after a motor vehicle accident, with multiple injuries and blood loss of more than 2 L. The blood urea and creatinine levels were both raised.
- In week 7, we had a patient with alcoholic liver cirrhosis, portal hypertension, portosystemic shunt and liver cell failure. His blood urea was below the normal range.
- In week 9, we had a patient presenting with chronic renal failure. His blood urea and creatinine were both raised.

These cases may trigger the following new questions:

- What do I know so far about blood urea and creatinine?
- What are the factors that could affect blood urea results?
- What are the scientific explanations for each of these differences?
- In this regard, what are the changes expected in a patient presenting with severe dehydration?
- Are there other relationships between these cases that could consolidate my understanding?

→ KEY 10 WHAT QUESTIONS MIGHT BE RAISED IN TUTORIAL 2?

Think about new questions that might be raised in the next tutorial. For example:
- What evidence do we have to support the final hypothesis?
- What evidence do we have against the other hypotheses?
- Are there any factors contributing to the patient's illness that we did not mention in our discussion in tutorial 1?
- Do we need to make any changes to our learning issues?
- How can we explain the patient's symptoms and signs?
- What types of investigation do we need? How can these investigations help us?
- What changes are expected in the results?
- What are our management goals and management plan? What factors can affect our management plan?
- What is the mechanism underlying the pathogenesis of the patient's symptoms, signs and investigation results?

→ KEY 11 HOW CAN NEW INFORMATION BE USED TO SOLVE NEW PROBLEMS?

Think about the use of information learnt for solving new problems. There may be three levels of difficulty in this approach because the problems:

1 are very similar to the problem you learnt but show a few differences, for example, demographic information, severity of symptoms, more clinical signs present, or
2 present with similar symptoms but the underlying structures and mechanisms involved are different. For example, you have studied a case of a patient with aortic stenosis: now try to use the knowledge learnt and work out new cases with other valvular problems such as aortic valve regurgitation or mitral stenosis, or
3 present with some of the symptoms you learnt but the history and clinical examination reveal that another body system is affected. For example, you have studied a case of a patient with aortic stenosis with shortness of breath: now try to apply your knowledge to another case with shortness of breath due to a respiratory problem such as chronic obstructive pulmonary disease.

What is the value of applying knowledge learnt to solve new problems? It will:
- allow you to learn the clinical significance of basic sciences
- deepen your understanding of the knowledge learnt and reinforce your memory
- show you how diseases can vary in severity and the way they present
- reinforce your problem-solving approach.

→ KEY 12 WHAT IS YOUR EVALUATION OF WHAT YOU HAVE LEARNT?

Think about the following self-evaluation questions:
- What are my areas of strength and areas needing improvement?
- Are there changes that I could make to improve my learning effectiveness?
- What skills would I like to develop to improve my performance?

- What type of assistance do I need to improve my performance?
- What goals am I interested in achieving this semester?
- How will I measure my progress toward these goals?

SELF-EVALUATION OF YOUR SELF-DIRECTED LEARNING SKILLS

Use the table opposite to evaluate your self-directed learning activities. Rate each criterion using a scale of 1 to 5, where 5 denotes the best ranking, 3 denotes not sure, 1 denotes not developed at all. Be fair in your ranking of each item. You can make copies of this table and use them to rank yourself every 3 months during the academic years, particularly in the first 2 years.

CONCLUSIONS

Problem-based learning cases provide students with the opportunity to define their learning needs and the areas they need to research to foster understanding of the problem discussed. Learning issues should: (1) reflect integrated knowledge from different disciplines, (2) be specific and clearly written as full sentences, (3) highlight specific objectives, (4) build on what the group knows, and (5) highlight knowledge of relevance to clinical practice. Learning issues may also highlight issues where students demonstrated misconception, incomplete understanding or disagreements. This chapter encourages you to learn from the common pitfalls most groups encounter in relation to learning issues. It also provides you with the keys for successful identification and preparation of your learning issues. It is important that each student research all the learning issues, not just one or two items so that in tutorial 2, members work together to construct the new information learnt and provide justification for issues raised in the case. To get the best out of this chapter, you need to put these keys into practice and use them regularly.

EVIDENCE-BASED LEARNING
Do student-defined learning issues increase quality and quantity of individual study?

An experiment was conducted in the context of a problem-based learning course to investigate the influence of a learning-goal-free problem scenario on the quality and quantity of individual study. In half of the tutorial groups, the problem scenario was constructed in such a way that it provided useful learning issues (goal-specified condition), whereas in the other half of the tutorial groups, the problem scenario did not provide learning issues (goal-free condition). It was demonstrated that students in the goal-free condition read more articles, studied longer, and spent more time reporting the studied literature than their peers in the goal-specified condition. These findings suggest that the use of goal-free problems has a positive effect on the students' individual study and the extensiveness of the tutorial group meeting.

Verkoeijen P, Rikers R, Winkel W, et al. Adv Health Sci Educ 2006; 11(4):337–347.
    Adapted with permission of the publisher.
For more information: http://www.springerlink.com/content/1573-1677/

CRITERION	RANKING				
	1	2	3	4	5
In tutorial 1, contributed to the case discussion that helped identify the learning issues					
In tutorial 1, contributed to the process of negotiating, amending and editing the final learning issues before leaving the tutorial					
On my own, demonstrated the ability to turn the learning issues into learning objectives and skills					
On my own, demonstrated the ability to plan my learning, use my self-directed learning model and apply my searching strategies					
On my own, demonstrated the ability to critically examine these resources					
On my own, demonstrated the ability to construct new information for each learning issue					
On my own, demonstrated the ability to manage my time in preparing the learning issues					
On my own, demonstrated the ability to think ahead about questions/issues that might be raised in tutorial 2					
In tutorial 2, demonstrated the ability to contribute to the discussion of these learning issues and construction of new information (answers) to the learning issue questions					
Other comments:					
What will you change in your self-directed learning next week to enhance your skills?					
What help do you need to enhance your self-directed learning?					
Who could help you?					

FURTHER READING
BOOKS

Long HB. Self-directed learning: Emerging theory and practice. Oklahoma City: Oklahoma Research Center for Continuing Professional and Higher Education; 1989.

Novak JD, Gowin DB. Learning how to learn. New York: Cambridge University Press; 1984.

ARTICLES AND RESEARCH PAPERS

Correa BB, Pinto PR, Rendas AB. How do learning issue relate with content in a problem-based learning pathophysiology course? Adv Physiol Educ 2003; 27(1-4):62–69.

Dolmans DH, Gijselaers WH, Schmidt HG, Van der Meer SB. Problem effectiveness in a course using problem-based learning. Acad Med 1993; 68:207–213.

Hueston WJ, Mallin R, Kern D. To what degree do problem-based learning issues change with clinical experience? Teach Learn Med 2002; 14(4):21-8-222.

Loyens S, Rikers R, Schmidt H. Students' concepts of constructivist learning: a comparison between a traditional and a problem-based learning curriculum. Adv Health Sci Educ Theory Prac 2006; 11(4):365–379.

Sigrell B, Sundblad G, Ronnas PA. To what extent do students generate learning issues that correspond to pre-set faculty objectives? Med Teach 2004; 26(4):378–380.

CHAPTER 6

Construction of mechanisms and flow charts

> And the actual achievements of biology are explanations in terms of mechanisms founded on physics and chemistry, which is not the same thing as explanations in terms of physics and chemistry.
>
> **MICHAEL POLANYI**

INTRODUCTION

An important aspect of problem-based learning (PBL), particularly in the early years of undergraduate medical and healthcare courses, is teaching basic sciences in a clinical format. Teaching in this format enhances students' skills in developing reasoning strategies, using information in relevant situations, generating hypotheses for problems identified and building mechanisms.

Mechanisms are flow charts illustrating a sequence of events. In simplified format they can be a sequence of events linked by arrows. Using mechanisms in a PBL curriculum allows students to use knowledge learnt and information provided in the case scenario—including psychosocial issues—to demonstrate how a suggested hypothesis might explain the patient's presenting problems. During this process, the group may discover they are unable to provide a thorough explanation and that they lack information in areas such as anatomy, biochemistry, microbiology, pathology, pathophysiology, pharmacology or physiology. The group might include these deficiencies in their knowledge in their *learning issues* list (see Ch 5).

However, building mechanisms is not an easy process and students often find it difficult to start their mechanisms or link mechanisms back to the information provided in the case scenario. Even in tutorial 2, after they have completed their learning issues and attended a few lectures, some groups struggle to build a good mechanism that links the information learnt to the pathophysiological processes, the patient's presenting symptoms and the clinical signs elicited in the case. Several factors can contribute to this difficulty:

- Early in a PBL course, students wonder what exactly constitutes a mechanism and how detailed their mechanisms should be.
- In high school, students are often trained to use rote learning rather than a learning style that encourages the application of knowledge, elaboration, reflection, critical thinking and integration.
- In PBL, many tutors are not experts in the disciplines related to the case. Despite their training in facilitating group discussion, some find it difficult to ask appropriate open-ended questions which enhance the discussion of mechanisms.
- Textbooks, lectures and other resources are usually discipline-based and do not help students integrate information as they create their mechanism.

- Building mechanisms requires a number of skills such as integration, deep understanding of basic sciences related to the case and the use of a logical flow.
- The group might find it difficult to convey to the scribe where the mechanism should start and how it should progress.
- There are no guidelines in training workshops or textbooks for students to assist them in understanding what constitutes a good mechanism.

WHY ARE MECHANISMS USEFUL IN TUTORIAL 1?

PBL cases are usually discussed in two, sometimes three, tutorials, depending on the structure of the curriculum. The educational objectives for creating diagrammatic mechanisms in tutorial 1 are not the same as those for developing a comprehensive mechanism in tutorial 2 (see Table 6.1).

TABLE 6.1 Mechanisms in PBL in tutorials 1 and 2: a comparison	
Tutorial 1	**Tutorial 2**
Students have no prior knowledge of the case and its contents	Students collect information from textbooks, online resources, lectures and practical classes related to their learning issues before attending the tutorial
Building a mechanism helps students identify areas of deficiency in their knowledge	Building a mechanism helps students integrate information learnt, apply knowledge and address patient's presentation and clinical signs
Mechanism may be broad and may include several hypotheses	Mechanism is usually focused on the final hypothesis
Mechanism is usually superficial, not detailed and may contain shortcuts	Mechanism is comprehensive, detailed and reflects integration of knowledge with no shortcuts

To understand more about the value of mechanisms in tutorial 1 let us use the case scenario below as an example.

Ms Linda Hart, a 42-year-old librarian, is brought to the emergency department at a local hospital by ambulance at 4 am. She is pale and vomiting fresh blood. Although drowsy, she is oriented and able to answer your questions. Ms Hart gives a history of vomiting large amounts of fresh blood at her house before arriving at the hospital. Last night, she started vomiting repeatedly after binge drinking. Thirty minutes later, the vomitus became bloody. Immediately on arrival to emergency the nurse tells you that Ms Hart's blood pressure is 100/60 mmHg (on lying flat), her pulse rate is 105/min and regular, her respiratory rate is 20/min and her temperature is 36.5°C. The registrar inserts a large intravenous line in her forearm vein and she is commenced on Haemaccel® intravenously. Ms Hart gives you a history of recurrent headaches, for which she takes aspirin tablets from time to time. Recently she has experienced abdominal pain and indigestion. Her bowels are regular but she has noticed that her motions have become black and soft over the last few hours. She has two tattoos on her back. She has been drinking a bottle of white wine a day for the last 10 years, but has increased her consumption since the death of her husband and son in a motor vehicle accident less than a year ago. As a result of her alcohol problem and feelings of depression, she was seen by a psychologist 6 months ago and was advised to attend counselling sessions regarding her alcohol problem. However, she has refused to attend.

Students identify haematemesis (vomiting blood) as one of the main problems. Their hypotheses for the problem are:
- Bleeding from an ulcer in the stomach (possibly caused by aspirin)
- Bleeding from the oesophagus (oesophageal varices)
- Bleeding from a tear in the oesophagus (caused by repeated vomiting)
- Bleeding from a cancer—oesophagus/stomach (cancers can ulcerate and bleed)

Because of uncertainty and lack of information, students can find it difficult to develop a mechanism explaining their hypotheses. They may develop a 'backward reasoning' approach. Using this approach, students begin by asking what could possibly cause Ms Hart to vomit up blood. They suggest, 'Bleeding from the oesophagus, stomach and duodenum'. Then they consider a new question: 'What causes bleeding from these structures? Is it mechanical damage to the lining tissues? Is it bleeding from abnormal blood vessels in the oesophagus or the stomach?' The scribe adds this new information to the whiteboard. As the group places these items in their mechanisms and thinks about the preceding question, they continue to develop their mechanism (Fig 6.1).

During this process, the group discovers that they lack information in four areas and they add them to their learning issues list: (1) What are the effects of excessive intake of alcohol? (2) Could the chronic intake of excessive alcohol cause these changes? (3) How does aspirin intake cause bleeding from the stomach? and (4) What caused these blood vessels to form? Note that groups vary in their approach; not all will use 'backward reasoning'.

Thus, the development of diagrammatic mechanisms in tutorial 1 is useful because it enables students to achieve the educational goals of:
- improving reasoning skills
- applying previously learnt information to a novel case
- identifying gaps in knowledge and defining learning issues
- prompting recognition of the need for a grasp of basic sciences to understand them in a clinical context
- fostering communication skills, peer–peer interaction and the ability to make links, use logic and clarify areas of confusion.

WHY ARE MECHANISMS USEFUL IN TUTORIAL 2?

By tutorial 2, students have researched their learning issues using textbooks, journal articles and appropriate websites, attended four or five lectures and possibly used a multimedia CD-ROM related to the case. They should be able to use and integrate information to build a comprehensive mechanism (Fig 6.2).

Therefore, the goals for developing mechanisms in tutorial 2 are to:
- integrate knowledge across disciplines and consider psychosocial issues in the case scenario
- allow students to appreciate the role of contributing factors and risk factors mentioned in the case history
- encourage reflection on the scientific basis of a patient's presenting problems, clinical signs and laboratory changes
- improve skills in organising pathophysiological changes at a body system and cellular level with no shortcuts.

It is a demanding task to achieve these goals so you should work effectively with your group to:

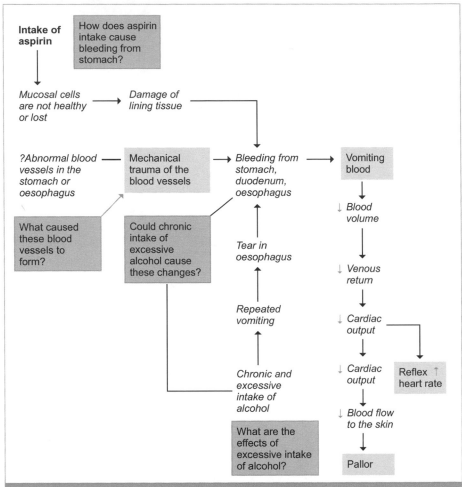

FIGURE 6.1 A mechanism developed in tutorial 1 to explain vomiting blood, increased heart rate and pallor.

1   construct mechanisms during the case discussion in tutorial 1 and again when you complete the whole case discussion
2   achieve the objectives of mechanisms in each of these tutorials
3   use knowledge gained from different resources such as textbooks, journal articles, and practical classes in an integrated way to build your mechanisms
4   evaluate your performance skills and participation to these processes.

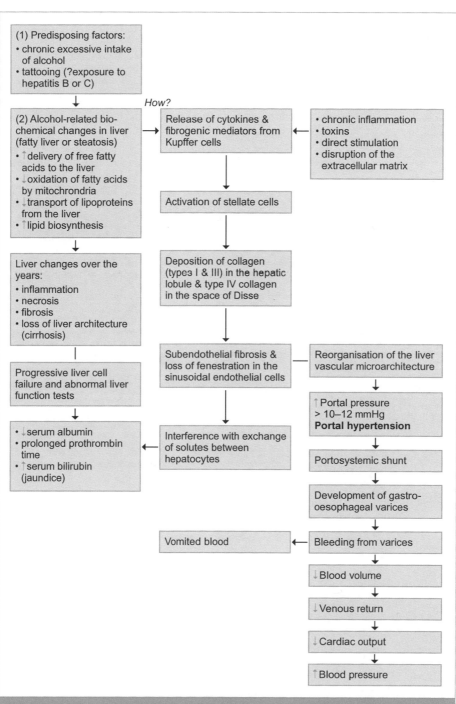

FIGURE 6.2 Mechanism created in tutorial 2.

USE OF CONCEPT MAPS IN KNOWLEDGE CONSTRUCTION

WHAT ARE CONCEPT MAPS?

Concept maps use networks to organise information. Networks comprise nodes (concepts) and links (to explain relationships between concepts). The concepts represent key information, causes, changes and subheads while the links may be uni- or bidirectional. Concepts and links are categorised or follow a particular order.

Concept maps are used to:
- organise and analyse information learnt
- clarify issues
- stimulate the generation of new ideas in a creative way
- apply knowledge learnt
- make the recall and review of information simpler
- encourage critical thinking
- accomplish meaningful learning
- help learners analyse and study relationships.

HOW DO CONCEPT MAPS AND MECHANISMS DIFFER?

Many students confuse concept maps and mechanisms. Some argue that mechanisms are a type of concept map and we do not need to make a comparison but my aim is to clarify differences between concept maps, as commonly used, and what we mean by mechanisms. This may also throw light on the structure of mechanisms and their uses in constructing pathogenesis and explaining different issues discussed in PBL cases. Table 6.2 (p. 100) summarises these differences.

KEYS FOR SUCCESSFUL FINAL MECHANISM WRITING

Many groups find it useful to construct a final mechanism summarising the whole case and work together with the help of a scribe to build their mechanism. Mechanisms may also be part of your written assessment, for example, as part of modified-essay questions and PBL-style questions. However, writing these mechanisms may be challenging for a number of reasons:
- There are no sources that guide learners on how to construct mechanisms.
- Most textbooks and other resources are discipline-based and do not present integrated knowledge.
- Construction of these mechanisms requires critical thinking, application of knowledge, and several other skills.

Before we start discussing the keys for successful mechanism writing, I would like you to think about the following case scenario and answer the question after the case. Then write down the processes and steps you used in constructing your mechanism. Once you finish, study the 12 keys for successful construction of mechanisms. To get the best out of this section, practise applying these steps and constructing mechanisms for the PBL cases you are studying in your course by using the 12 keys.

What are the major categories of concept maps?

Flow chart concept map

Description: Organises information in a linear way using arrows. Usually the arrows are pointed in the same direction.

Uses: This type of concept map can be used in: (1) illustrating a sequence of events, (2) demonstrating relationships, for example, cause–effect relationships, (3) showing temporal changes, for example, the steps in a PBL discussion in tutorial 1 and the time allocated for each step, and (4) decision-making strategies and simple management protocols.

Hierarchy concept map

Description: Organises information in descending order of significance. The most significant item is placed at the top of the map. This is usually one item only and it leads to other items of less significance.

Uses: This type of concept map can be used in: (1) classification and creation of taxonomy, (2) organisation of a body system, and (3) organisational structure.

Image-based concept map

Description: Organises information by using an image or illustration related to the concept discussed.

Uses: This type of concept map can be used in: (1) parasitology, for example, showing the malaria cycle in the human body and the changes in the parasite in the liver and red blood cells, and (2) physiology, for example, the bilirubin metabolism and how the liver cells (hepatocytes) handle bilirubin.

Multidimensional concept map

Description: Organises information and state of information in a simple two- or three-dimensional map.

Uses: This type of concept map can be used in: (1) demonstrating complex structures that have several interactive components, and (2) basic sciences, for example, showing factors affecting the solubility of bile.

Spider concept map (mind map)

Description: Organises information by placing a main 'theme' also known as 'main items' or 'topic title' in the centre of the map while all subheads are placed on the periphery extending from, or on one side of, the centre of the map.

Uses: This type of concept map can be used in: (1) a brainstorming exercise, for example, possible causes of the patient's problem, contributing factors or differential diagnosis, (2) showing categories, and (3) summarising key points related to a theme.

Systems concept map

Description: Organises information in a format similar to a flow chart with additional 'input' and 'output'.

Uses: This type of concept map can be used in: (1) metabolic cycles, for example, urea cycle, citric acid cycle, and (2) physiological cycles, for example, blood circulation.

There are a number of computer programs you can use to construct your concept maps. One of these programs is the CmapTools which allows users to construct and navigate their own concept maps. The CmapTools software is free to download and install in your computer. The website is http://cmap.ihmc.us/download/

TABLE 6.2 Key similarities and differences between concept maps and mechanisms

Features	Concept maps	Mechanisms
Key similarities	Organise information Summarise key points Provide an easy-to-read and remember summary May focus on a number of concepts and how they are related	Organise information Summarise key points Provide an easy-to-read and remember summary Usually focus on explanations of one concept or more
Key differences Purpose	Brainstorming Categorisation Showing hierarchy Organising knowledge learnt	Progress/changes over time and of underlying processes Basic sciences behind the changes Interpretation of findings Justification Role of contributing factors and the role of psychosocial issues
Nature	Static Lists Main items and sub-items	Dynamic Sequence of events and changes over time
Knowledge	Knowledge integrated Do not necessarily provide explanations or justifications	Knowledge integrated across disciplines Provide explanations and justifications Tell a story Information organised: (1) contributing factors, (2) body and, (3) target issues
Outcomes for the learner	Improve learning Organise information	Enhances: — learning — cognitive skills — deep understanding, integration and construction of new information

CASE SCENARIO

Michael Panagopoulos is an 18-year-old tourist from Greece. Two months after his arrival in Australia he develops a wound infection and is seen by a GP. His wound is cleaned and he is prescribed an antibiotic. Over the next few days he experiences pain and his wound is healing well, but he feels very tired. He comes in again to see the GP because he has developed shortness of breath when he walks a short distance. His girlfriend also notices that his eyes are yellowish in colour. Michael has no fever and his wound is healing well. Further history reveals that he has no history of medical illness or hospital treatment but does have a family history of anaemia. On examination, he looks pale. His pulse is 110/min (normal: 60–100/min), blood pressure 110/70 mmHg (normal: 100/60–130/80 mmHg), respiratory rate 20/min (normal: 12–16/min) and temperature 36.8°C (normal: 36.6–37.2°C). The sclerae of his eyes look yellow. No changes in the colour of his urine.

Using your knowledge of basic and clinical sciences, describe the most likely mechanism by which Michael developed the symptoms of tiredness, shortness of breath, pallor, jaundice and rapid pulse rate. Your answer should explain each of Michael's symptoms. You may use a flow diagram to outline your answer.

The following keys will help you create a balanced and integrated mechanism.

→ KEY 1 GENERATE HYPOTHESES

Before you start building your mechanism, you need to be sure of the focus and scope of your mechanism. This is particularly important for mechanisms you are developing with your group at the end of the case or mechanisms you are asked to develop in the summative examination. Your starting point is to identify possible hypotheses for the patient's problems. You may have identified the following to explain Michael's tiredness, shortness of breath, pallor, jaundice and rapid pulse rate:

1 Infection/antibiotic-associated haemolysis (this is likely to occur in patients with glucose-6-phosphate dehydrogenase deficiency).
2 Antibiotic-associated suppression of his bone marrow (stopped the production of red blood cells, white blood cells and platelets but it does not explain his jaundice).
3 Septicaemia (but this is unlikely because Michael has no history of fever or rigors, his haemodynamics are stable, he has no pain and the wound is healing well).
4 Liver toxicity caused by antibiotics (this may explain his jaundice but not other symptoms).

→ KEY 2 MAKE A FOCUS

Refining your hypotheses is the next logical step. Your aim is to weigh the evidence for and against each hypothesis and decide on your final hypothesis. The first hypothesis is the most likely. Jaundice means that there is excess bilirubin deposited in the sclerae. This could be the consequence of haemolysis: decreased oxygen-carrying capacity of red blood cells, shortness of breath, rapid pulse and tiredness. Michael has no evidence of septicaemia, hepatocellular toxicity or obstructive jaundice.

As you refine your hypothesis, consider the following key questions:
- Is this an acute, chronic or recurrent problem?
- Are the patient's symptoms and signs due to local and/or systemic problems?
- Are the patient's problems due to physiological or pathological changes?
- What are the pathophysiological processes responsible for the patient's problems? (for example, inflammation, degeneration, trauma, mechanical, immunological, neoplasia, toxicity, necrosis, hypertrophy, atrophy)
- Which body systems, organs, structures are involved?
- What supportive evidence do we have from the patient's symptoms and signs?
- What further information do we need to support our final hypothesis?
- How have the laboratory investigations and other investigations assisted us?

→ KEY 3 EXAMINE YOUR FINAL HYPOTHESIS

What I mean by 'Examine your final hypothesis' is:
1 Examine each piece of your supportive evidence.

2 Expand your thoughts and reflections on your justification.

3 Think about the pathophysiological changes associated with your final hypothesis.

Examination of the final hypothesis shows:

- The changes in the colour of Michael's sclerae occurred after the intake of antibiotic.
- Bilirubin is a pigment. It is the end-product of haemoglobin and is able to stain the sclerae of eyes yellowish when present in excess.
- Michael's tiredness, rapid pulse and shortness of breath occurred after the intake of antibiotics and these symptoms can be due to acute haemolysis (anaemia).
- There is no evidence of acute hepatic injury, septicaemia or obstructive jaundice.
- Michael has a family history of anaemia.
- Michael is from Greece (up to 30% of people, particularly males, from the Mediterranean area, have glucose-6-phosphate dehydrogenase deficiency).
- It is most likely that Michael has glucose-6-phosphate dehydrogenase deficiency and developed acute haemolysis, triggered by infection and/or the antibiotic.

→ KEY 4 LIST KEYWORDS/CONCEPTS

Before you start constructing your mechanism think about these seven key questions. As you study each question, write down the keywords you would use to address each of these questions and which you could use in constructing your mechanism:

1 What are the key issues you would like to include in your mechanism?

2 What are the factors contributing to Michael's problems?

3 Are there any genetic or environmental triggers for these problems? What are the key issues here?

4 What are the initial physiological, biochemical or pathological changes responsible for these problems? What are the keywords and scientific terms related to these changes?

5 Following the initial changes, are there any subsequent changes I could include?

6 What body systems, organs, structures, cells are involved in these changes?

7 What are the pathological processes behind these changes (inflammation, trauma, mechanical, immunological, neoplasia, toxicity, necrosis, hypertrophy, atrophy)?

Examples of keywords you might come up with for Michael's case:

Haemolysis
Glucose-6-phosphate dehydrogenase deficiency
Glutathione
Cell membrane
Oxidants
Oxidative stress
X chromosome
Antibiotics
Inheritance
Anaemia
Decrease in oxygen-carrying capacity
Exchange of gases in alveoli (lungs)
Excessive loss of haemoglobin from red blood cells
Normal half-life of red blood cells
Circulation
Bilirubin pigment

Tiredness
Biliverdin
Bilirubin binds to albumin
Liver
Uptake of bilirubin
More bilirubin in the circulation
Liver capacity
Unconjugated bilirubin
Sclerae of eyes
Staining
Yellowish colouration
Less oxygen carried to muscles
Less oxygen carried to body cells
Less metabolic process
Tiredness, fatigue
Less fuel available to produce energy
Reflex stimulation of respiration
Sympathetic stimulation
Rapid pulse
Cardiac output
Rapid circulation
Fewer red blood cells in capillaries (pallor)

→ KEY 5 PLAN YOUR MECHANISM

Planning your mechanism is the key for creating a well-structured and balanced mechanism. Your planning should aim to:
- construct a balanced mechanism conveying the big picture and fine details
- use knowledge from basic sciences to explain the patient's symptoms and signs
- organise the flow of the different components of your mechanism
- present information logically to reinforce meaningful learning and critical thinking
- show deep understanding of the concepts addressed in the mechanism
- accommodate different components of the mechanism (for example, contributing factors, pathophysiological changes, consequences, justification) in an integrated manner.

→ KEY 6 START WITH CONTRIBUTING FACTORS

One of the stages that is often missing in mechanisms is addressing contributing factors for the patient's problems that are directly related to the final hypothesis. Contributing factors are usually provided in the case scenario. They may include:

Environmental factors
Occupational exposure and risks
Genetic background and family history
Exposure to infectious agents
Travel overseas
Hobbies, tattooing
Trauma, injuries, fractures
Smoking, illicit drug use, alcohol intake

Risk factors for vascular problems, e.g. obesity, high blood pressure, high blood cholesterol/triglycerides, family history, diabetes

Medications, allergies

Psychosocial issues

Age, gender and patient's background

Previous illnesses

In Michael's case, the following contributing factors may be considered: (1) being a young male from Greece, (2) wound infection and intake of antibiotics, (3) family history of anaemia (? glucose-6-phosphate dehydrogenase deficiency).

→ KEY 7 ENSURE YOUR MECHANISM REFLECTS KNOWLEDGE INTEGRATION

One of the main aims of your mechanism is to demonstrate your ability to integrate knowledge learnt from a wide range of resources with your final hypothesis. This should be reflected in the keywords and concepts you have identified and in the way you present these concepts in the mechanism. Disciplines may include anatomy, biochemistry, genetics, histology, immunology, medicine, microbiology, paediatrics, pathology, pharmacology, physiology and psychology. Some cases may raise public health issues or ethical and moral issues.

→ KEY 8 ADDRESS BODY SYSTEM, ORGAN, CELLULAR AND MOLECULAR LEVELS

The pathophysiological changes you will include in your mechanism should be explained in a meaningful way. This may necessitate discussion of the changes at body system, organ, cellular and molecular levels. Most mechanisms will require this level of detail. However, if your mechanism is part of a summative examination question, you need to read the question and assess what exactly is needed from you. One clue for you is the marks or time allocated for the question. If 5 or 6 marks are allocated for the question, you do not need to include such details. Do not make your mechanism overcrowded; one or two important cellular changes may be enough.

→ KEY 9 PROVIDE AN EXPLANATION FOR PATIENT'S SYMPTOMS AND SIGNS

The objectives of your mechanism may include explanations for the patient's symptoms and signs. This part of your mechanism should:
* explain the scientific basis behind each of the patient's symptoms and signs
* highlight any relationships between the patient's presenting symptoms
* address pathological processes underlying the patient's symptoms and signs.

→ KEY 10 PROVIDE AN EXPLANATION FOR INVESTIGATION RESULTS

The aim of your mechanism may also be to provide an explanation of the results of investigations. This component of your mechanism could include:
* changes in biochemical tests
* histological and cytological changes
* radiological imaging changes (for example, CT and MRI scans, echocardiogram, nuclear medicine studies, ultrasound, X-ray)

- electrocardiography changes
- haematological changes.

    You may address:
- nature of changes
- basic sciences behind these changes
- consequences that may result from these changes.

→ KEY 11 ENSURE THERE ARE NO SHORTCUTS

How would you discover areas with shortcuts in your mechanism? Ask yourself these questions as you review your mechanism:
- Are there areas that can be better explained in my mechanism?
- Are there any other concepts I could add to provide a more meaningful understanding of the pathogenesis of the condition?
- Will the new information explain things better?

→ KEY 12 REVIEW AND AMEND

Consider the following points as you review and amend your mechanism:
- illogical flow
- unclear issues
- crowded and unbalanced areas
- contradictions
- areas that can be improved
- new information to be added
- redundant information to be omitted
- incorrect and poor links between concepts
- targets you were asked to address in your mechanism.

EXERCISES

Here are some exercises to test your understanding of the keys. I have provided a model answer to Exercise 2.

Exercise 1
Use the 12 keys to improve the mechanism below.

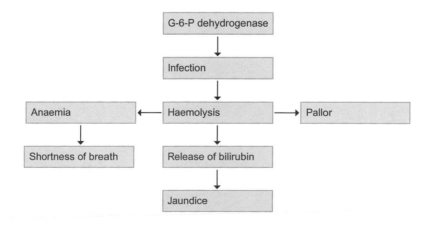

Exercise 2

Use the key concepts below to construct a mechanism for Michael's case. The aim is to use boxes, organise information and show links.

A model answer

Michael possibly has glucose-6-phosphate dehydrogenase deficiency (G-6-PD D), the gene is located on the X chromosome ⇨ this defect affects carbohydrate metabolism (the hexose-monophosphate shunt) ⇨ failure of reduced glutathione (GSH) production (normally responsible for stability of haemoglobin and red cell membrane).

Now the presence of bacterial infection + oxidants (antibiotic) ⇨ increases the likelihood of damage to the red cell membrane (due to a lack of reduced GSH) ⇨ disturbance of patient's red blood cells' membranes ⇨ haemolysis of a significant number of patient's red blood cells (RBCs) (the normal half-life of RBCs is 120 days, they are normally damaged by macrophages in the spleen, liver and marrow) ⇨ release of large amounts of haemoglobin into the circulation (more than the capacity of the liver, which is normally responsible for handling haemoglobin) ⇨ the released haemoglobin is broken down into two main components (globin and haeme portion) ⇨ the haeme portions are broken down into iron (Fe^{3+}) and biliverdin (a greenish pigment) ⇨ biliverdin is reduced to bilirubin ⇨ bilirubin binds to albumin, a carrier protein, and is transported in the blood to the liver cells (hepatocytes) ⇨ the liver cells take up bilirubin and bilirubin is conjugated in liver cells ⇨ conjugated bilirubin is water soluble and is secreted into bile ⇨ but in his condition, large amounts of unconjugated bilirubin are accumulated in patient's blood as well ⇨ unconjugated bilirubin increases in patient's circulation ⇨ excess bilirubin precipitated in the elastic tissues of the sclerae of the eyes.

Excessive haemolysis of red blood cells ⇨ decreased red blood cell number ⇨ decreased oxygen-carrying capacity of haemoglobin ⇨ poor exchange of gases in alveoli and less delivery of oxygen needed to produce energy in different body cells ⇨ tiredness.

Also the decreased availability of oxygen to brain cells contributes to this tiredness.

Because of decreased oxygen concentration in his blood ⇨ reflex stimulation and sympathetic activation ⇨ increased nerve impulses through the sympathetic supply to the heart ⇨ tachycardia (increased heart rate) and rapid circulation to compensate for the lack of oxygen.

Also reflex stimulation to the respiratory centre in the medulla oblongata and increased sympathetic stimulation to the respiratory system ⇨ increased breathing rate on mild exercise (a sense of shortness of breath).

You might use a diagram to outline your mechanism (see Fig 6.3).

CONCLUSIONS

Developing diagrammatic mechanisms in PBL tutorials offers a number of educational benefits. The educational objectives achieved by developing mechanisms in tutorial 1 differ from those achieved in tutorial 2. In tutorial 1 you should be improving your reasoning skills; learning to apply previously learnt information

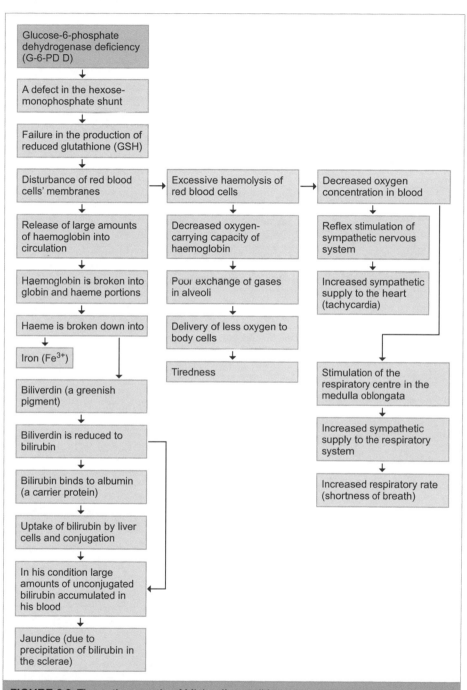

FIGURE 6.3 The pathogenesis of Michael's condition.

to a novel case and to identify areas of deficiency in knowledge and define your learning issues; understanding the need for a grasp of basic sciences and improving your communication skills in the group. In tutorial 2 the aim is to integrate your knowledge across disciplines and understand the significance of psychosocial issues in the case scenario. You need to consider the role of contributing factors and risk factors mentioned in the case history. You also need to reflect on the scientific basis of a patient's presenting problems, clinical signs and laboratory changes and to improve your skills in organising pathophysiological changes at a body system and cellular level with no shortcuts. The use of the 12 keys offers a good opportunity for you to write integrated, balanced and meaningful mechanisms.

FURTHER READING
BOOKS
Jonassen DH, Beissner K, Yacci MA. Structural knowledge. Techniques for conveying, assessing, and acquiring structural knowledge. Hillsdale, NJ: Lawrence Erlbaum Associates, 1993.

Novak JD, Gowin DB. Learning how to learn. New York: Cambridge University Press; 1984.

ARTICLES AND RESEARCH PAPERS
Azer SA. Facilitation of students' discussion in problem-based learning tutorials to create mechanisms: the use of five key questions. AnnAcad Medicine Singapore 2005; 34(8):492–498.

Guerrero AP. Mechanistic case diagramming: a tool for problem-based learning. Acad Med 2001; 76(4):385–389.

Novak JD. Clarity with concept maps: a tool for students and teachers alike. Sci Teach 1991; 58(7):45–49.

Novak, JD. How do we learn our lesson? Taking students through the process. Sci Teach 1993; 60(3):51–55.

CHAPTER 7

Effective use of learning resources

All men by nature desire to know   **ARISTOTLE**

INTRODUCTION

Finding the resources you need for your learning is one of the keys for success. More important is how to use these resources effectively and build on existing knowledge. With the current explosion of scientific and medical knowledge and the availability of electronic resources, finding information is not difficult. The widespread dissemination of scientific, medical and health information and easy access to this information has made major changes to the learner's priorities. The challenges now are: how to select the best resources you need, how to use the new information in answering your questions and how the new knowledge fits with what you already know.

In a problem–based learning (PBL) curriculum there is a strong emphasis on the patient and patient-centred care. So, as you select your resources, it is very important to think about basic sciences related to the case and to give priority to the patient. Your goal is not just collecting information about medical sciences. You need to think about the bioethical, psychosocial and cultural issues in the case that can add to your understanding of the problem. Use appropriate resources covering these areas to foster your humanity and communication skills and your understanding of behavioural medicine, the psychology of illness and social issues.

In addition to the resources you find in these areas (see Appendices A and B), I suggest you read books that deal with the patient, doctors' stories, the work of general practitioners, biographies of patients, stories of sickness and emerging ethical issues. This reading will broaden your understanding of medicine and the range of issues you need to consider in your learning. See the 'Wider reading' box on the next page. While I recommend you read these books and articles, your main resource remains the subject guide provided by your school. You should read it as you commence your course and keep a copy handy for reference throughout the year.

SUBJECT GUIDES

A *subject guide* is an aid, prepared by the course coordinators and the faculty education unit to help students manage their learning. It is usually in the form of a printed or an electronic document that can be downloaded from the faculty website. The subject guide provides:
* the framework of the course and overall philosophy of the curriculum
* themes and objectives of the course
* educational and online resources

Wider reading
Books
Hawkins AH. Reconstructing illness: studies in pathography. West Lafyette, Indiana: Purdue University Press; 1993.
Kushner TK, Thomasma DC, eds. Ward ethics. Dilemmas for medical students and doctors in training. Cambridge: Cambridge University Press; 2001.
Toombs SK. The meaning of illness: A phenomenological account of the different perspectives of physician and patient. Boston: Kluwer; 1992.
Articles
Jones AH. Narrative in medical ethics. West J Med. 1999; 171(1):50–52. Online. Available: www.pubmedcentral.nih.gov/articlerender.fcgi?artid=1305740
Tomlin PJ. A memorable incident: When is a spade not a spade? BMJ 1999; 318(7178):256. Online: available: www.bmj.bmjjournals.com/cgi/reprint/318/7178/256.pdf
Maguire P, Pitceathly C. Key communication skills and how to acquire them. BMJ 2002; 325(7366): 697–700.

- a management tool to help students organise their self-directed learning and use their time effectively
- strategies for using learning resources, searching for information, asking open-ended questions and applying information learnt to solve new problems
- help for students in adopting a learning style to suit the curriculum and their learning needs. For example, in a PBL course students will need to adopt a learning style that fosters their self-directed learning and collaborative learning.

In most PBL courses, cases are not released to the students in the subject guide at the beginning of the year. Cases are released on a weekly basis: students do not receive information in advance about the case objectives. The only clue they have is the body systems addressed in the semester or during the year. However, in *hybrid PBL courses* (courses that use a mix of PBL and other learning approaches) and those using a case-based approach, students may be given the cases at the beginning of each semester.

MAIN TOPICS COVERED IN THE SUBJECT GUIDE

Subject guides may cover the following topics:
- overall objectives and outcomes of the course
- the philosophy of the curriculum and its rationale
- the timetable
- contact details for student support, staff contacts, academic mentors and the course coordinators
- assessment objectives, types of assessment tool and examples, competencies to be examined, distribution of marks, dates for formative and summative assessment
- recommended multimedia, textbooks and online resources
- keys for learning approaches and tips on how to get the best from your course
- useful resources on learning, for example, tips on successful discussion in PBL tutorials.

EFFECTIVE USE OF YOUR SUBJECT GUIDE

- Make yourself familiar with the subject guide at the start of the academic year.
- Highlight key information you might need to refer to during the year.
- Read the learning outcomes and overall objectives of the course.
- Write your reflections and plans in your reflective journal (see Ch 9).
- Start planning for adopting a learning style that corresponds with the PBL philosophy. You do not need to write any details at this stage. You will be able to add thoughts/actions to your reflective journal as the course progresses and you understand more about your priorities and needs.
- Orient yourself to different resources that you might use.
- Organise your computer files (see Ch 8).
- Keep your subject guide (and future guides) together with this book; you will need to use them throughout the first 2 years.

LEARNING STYLES AND LEARNING RESOURCES

A number of researchers have identified the following learning styles used by students using learning resources:

1 *Superficial learners.* The learners in this group:
   — concentrate on memorising facts with little understanding
   — do not apply knowledge learnt to real-life problems
   — fail to realise the key principles behind the knowledge they acquire
   — treat tasks as an external imposition
   — do not link new information learnt to what they already know
   — are less likely than their peers to use several resources as they search for their learning issues.

2 *Deep learners.* The learners in this group:
   — try to understand what is behind the words. Give understanding a priority
   — always define concepts and principles learnt
   — tend to construct information acquired from a number of resources
   — understand the relationship between concepts and make connections in the knowledge encountered
   — build new knowledge acquired on existing knowledge base
   — tend to integrate information learnt
   — focus on concepts and principles when they work on a new problem
   — ask themselves questions to focus on in their search for new information
   — think about new questions as they come across new knowledge
   — weigh evidence collected to support their views
   — are able to analyse new information and make conclusions.

3 *Strategic learners.* The learners in this group:
   — are motivated by achievements and adopt strategies to achieve their goals
   — organise their time and plan their learning
   — are clear about the goals and objectives of the curriculum and subsequent assessment
   — study information provided by their schools about assessment—competencies to be tested, tools to be used and overall assessment structure

— use feedback provided by their tutors to improve their learning and attitudes
— focus on key principles and core curriculum
— use earlier examinations to predict questions.

4   *Life-long learners.* The learners in this group possess most of the qualities mentioned under deep and strategic learners. Moreover, they possess these qualities:
   — plan ahead for future learning
   — are passionate about learning new skills and acquiring new knowledge
   — use learning resources effectively
   — reflect on what they learn and tend to share knowledge learnt with others
   — demonstrate educability—the capability of being educated.

5   *Innovative learners.* These learners are able to create something new. They make changes to the profession by bringing something new and useful to our community. The history of medicine is filled with examples of medical students who have made discoveries during their undergraduate study.

RESOURCES IN PROBLEM-BASED LEARNING COURSES

In a PBL curriculum you will need to use several resources to construct your learning issues and deepen your understanding. This might be challenging for you in the first weeks of your first year and there could be a number of reasons for your concern. Students whom I have taught in PBL courses exhibited their concern by asking questions such as:

'I never used to study from several resources in my high school.'
'I used to study one text for each subject.'
'Books are not integrated and now I need to integrate knowledge and construct new information for my learning issues.'
'I am not sure how I can use several resources at the same time.'
'How much time should I spend on my self-directed learning?'
'How will I review for examinations? Will I read everything again before examinations?'
'How should I select my resources? Is there any way to identify good resources?'
'How can I use these resources to prepare my learning issues?'
'Will I be able to remember information from all these resources?'
'What should I do to master this skill?'

You may have similar questions. Some of the questions were answered in Chs 4 and 5. In this chapter I provide more detail and show you how using several resources is a skill you can develop. Before we start, let me remind you of some of the benefits of using several resources in preparing your learning issues:

• Some concepts are difficult to understand; by using several resources you will discover new dimensions of the issue and this will facilitate your understanding.
• You are able to see relationships, for example, structure and function of cells and body organs; normal functions and progress of pathological processes.
• You are able to examine different aspects of a problem.
• You are able to provide justification for your views.
• Resources will not all provide you with the same thing. Some will provide you with knowledge and detail; others will provide you with three-dimensional models, animations and clinical application or self-assessment questions. By using

different resources you will be confident about your preparation, able to discuss issues to the depth required and structure and encode information learnt in meaningful ways (form a schema). This will enhance long-term retention of the information you have acquired.

LEARNING SCHEMA

A learning *schema* is the process of constructing information in a meaningful way to facilitate its storage. Information needs to be encoded in order to be remembered and recalled. This building process is enhanced when the acquired knowledge:
- is constructed by the learner
- is linked to existing knowledge
- is structured in an organised, logical and meaningful way
- answers the learner's questions
- is comprised of clinical applications
- provides explanations and interpretations of the findings.

The point I make here is that the number of resources to be used is not the key for achieving deep and strategic learning. What is more important is intelligent use of the resources by understanding their use and which will suit your learning style. Here is a list of resources you could use in your PBL curriculum:
- textbooks
- electronic textbooks
- journal and review articles
- PBL cases
- educational websites
- lecture notes
- lecturers' PowerPoints
- interactive multimedia
- medical dictionary
- anatomy atlas
- pharmacology and therapeutic handbook
- clinical examination videos or DVDs
- interactive bank of questions
- knowledge you construct during your self-directed learning and your own notes
- your group discussion summaries
- patient educational resources (e.g. websites, booklets, pamphlets)
- clinical rounds
- reflective journals/portfolios
- practical classes and faculty subject guides
- recorded lectures and seminars
- student management system
- cadaver, pre-dissected specimens, pathology specimens
- your own notes and summaries from lectures.

There are vast treasures of databases to help you find appropriate research and review papers accessible by computer. For instance, the MEDLINE database contains more than 11 million biographic citations in medical and life sciences from over 7300 international biomedical journals. To benefit from the following section you should have already developed computer skills such as accessing the internet and using email.

The US National Library of Medicine (NLM) is responsible for the free availability of medical knowledge from MEDLINE to everyone with internet access. MEDLINE is derived from the Index Medicus which began in 1879. The NLM first used computers in 1964 to prepare the Index Medicus for printing. In 1971, online searching of the MEDLINE database was introduced. In 1986, Grateful Med (since phased out) was introduced to permit searching MEDLINE directly from personal computers. Since then other databases have evolved to serve medical, healthcare and biomedical professionals and students. Table 7.1 summarises the commonly used databases.

WHY IS RESEARCHING THE LITERATURE USEFUL?

Literature research allows you to:
- gain up-to-date knowledge in a particular area
- develop deep understanding
- fill the gaps in textbooks and other resources
- use evidence-based practices
- develop your self-directed learning skills
- learn how to interpret results and assess the significance of research outcomes.

LIMITATIONS OF JOURNAL ARTICLES AND LITERATURE REVIEWS

- Issues are too specialised and may be written about at a level of detail greater than needed in undergraduate courses. The focus is usually narrow and deep so does not show the breadth needed in PBL.
- Issues may be focused on either the basic or the clinical sciences related to a topic. There is no opportunity to see the relationship between the two.
- Results of the studies may not be supported by other researchers and the views presented in the paper may be controversial.
- Reviews are usually long and reading them can be time consuming.
- The methodology used in most research papers is often complex and difficult to understand. The statistical approaches and interpretation of the results may add to this complexity. This is particularly challenging to first-year students with limited knowledge of research methodology, statistical analysis and data interpretation. To overcome this challenge, most PBL courses provide students in their first year with journal articles appropriate to their needs. However, as students progress, they are left on their own to select the papers and reviews they need for their learning.
- In some review papers the issues discussed are theoretical and do not help students refine their hypotheses or reach clear, meaningful learning objectives.

WHAT ARE THE AIMS OF LITERATURE SEARCH?

From the perspective of a PBL student, the main aim of the literature search is to enhance your knowledge about the subject areas and fill the gaps in your knowledge. A literature search allows you to practise the exercise of independent critical evaluation of published papers and selection of appropriate papers to foster your learning. This is an essential component of your self-directed learning skill development. As you progress you will need to look at evidence-based practices for your management

TABLE 7.1 Databases commonly used by medical, healthcare and biomedical professionals

Database	Provider	Access	URL	Comments
PubMed	The US National Medical Library and the National Institutes of Health	Free	http://www.ncbi.nlm.nih.gov/	Search items may be: — topic — author, or — journal
HighWire	Stanford University's High Wire Press	Free	http://highwire.stanford.edu/	HighWire hosts the largest repository of free-text, peer-reviewed content, with over 1000 journals and more than 4,300,000 free full-text articles online. With various partners HighWire produces 71 of the 200 most frequently cited journals.
OVID	Wolters Kluwer, Amsterdam	Membership required	http://www.ovid.com/sites/index.jsp	OVID is a globally focused information provider, founded in 1988. In the US it is used in 93% of medical libraries and 97% of teaching hospitals. OVID offers clinicians, professionals, students and researchers in the medical, scientific and academic fields customisable solutions of content and services.
Google Scholar	Google	Free	http://scholar.google.com/	Provides a simple way to broadly search for scholarly literature. You can search across many disciplines and sources: peer-reviewed papers, theses, books, abstracts and articles, from academic publishers, professional societies, preprint repositories, universities and other scholarly organisations.

options. This area is usually deficient in most textbooks and reviewing the literature (e.g. the Cochrane Collaboration and the Cochrane Library—http://www.cochrane. org/reviews/clibintro.htm) will provide you with more information about: (1) type and level of evidence available, (2) studies undertaken to assess evidence, (3) helping the patient decide, and (4) changes in your practices as a result of the evidence.

Searching the literature will also help you to:

- learn the current understanding of particular concepts and research issues
- understand that differences between studies may be the result of different research design, methodology and underlying conditions
- learn how to distinguish between different views on a research issue and your own opinion
- learn how to justify your views.

SUCCESSFUL LITERATURE SEARCH

Before you start searching, orient yourself to the different literature databases. For example, you could read PubMed Help available at http://www.ncbi.nlm.nih.gov/ books/bv.fcgi?rid=helppubmed.chapter.pubmedhelp and PubMed Online Training, PubMed Tutorial, available at http://www.nlm.nih.gov/bsd/disted/pubmed.html. Table 7.2 provides step-by-step search actions for the PubMed database.

EFFECTIVE USE OF MEDICAL DICTIONARIES

Medical and healthcare dictionaries are among the most essential resources you need in PBL tutorials. Most of the universities that have adopted PBL as a teaching approach provide each PBL room with a set of resources and textbooks. These resources include a medical and healthcare dictionary, anatomy atlas, drug and therapeutic resource as well as a set of textbooks (see Appendix B for more detail). Some universities also provide electronic versions of these resources in PBL rooms. Your tutor will encourage you to use the dictionary once you encounter a new medical or scientific term. You may need to discuss the meaning of the term and link the information learnt with the case scenario. Medical dictionaries can provide you with a wide range of information; not just the definition or the uses of medical terms. The benefits of using medical dictionaries in PBL tutorials can be summarised as:

- understanding the use of new terms in relation to the case scenario as well as other common uses
- understanding the origin of the term (this is its etymology)
- depending on the term you are looking for, understanding the anatomical, physiological, pathological, biochemical, histological, immunological, microbiological, pharmacological or toxicological information related to the case
- information provided by the dictionary may open the door for new terms and further information related to the topic discussed
- diagrams or illustrations provided will help you to see other dimensions to the information provided, not just the meaning of the term
- in many instances the clinical applications or signs, symptoms and complications of a condition related to a term are provided
- most medical dictionaries provide a pronunciation guide, presentation of plurals, internationally used abbreviations, cross references and synonymous terms.

Table 7.3 summarises the commonly used medical dictionaries in medical and healthcare PBL courses. The *Mosby's*, *Dorland's Illustrated* and *Stedman's* dictionaries

TABLE 7.2 Step-by-step search actions of PubMed database

Step	Example	Actions	What you should do	What you should not do
1. Identify key concepts in your research question.	Write the keywords for, say: 'pathogenesis of aortic stenosis'.	Keywords are: 'pathogenesis' 'aortic stenosis'. Enter the words into the search box. Press ENTER or GO.	Link terms with special words AND, OR and NOT in capital letters. Use quotations to unite words into phrases that can be searched as if they were a single word.	If you enter 'pathogenesis AND aortic stenosis', you may retrieve over 10,000 citations and if you enter 'pathogenesis AND aortic AND stenosis', the search turns up more than 9000 citations (i.e. is more focused on your topic).
2. Use asterisk character (*) as a wild card.	Search for pathogenesis.	Keyword is 'pathogenesi*'. Press ENTER or GO.	The use of the asterisk (*) will direct the search to find articles that match the term as spelled up to the point of the asterisk, regardless of the letters that follow. This search will include 'pathogenesis' 'pathogenesin' 'pathogenesic' and 'pathogenesity'.	This type of search is needed for special research reasons. It will not help you in a PBL search.
3. Search by author.	Search papers authored by John A Smith.	Keywords are: 'Smith JA'.	Type 'Smith JA'. Click the limit tab to use 'Author' search only. Or you could type 'Smith JA [au]'.	The following entries will not help you: 'Smith John' or 'John A Smith'.
4. Search by journal title.	Search the issues of Medical Teacher.	Keyword: 'Medical Teacher'.	Enter in the search box either full title: 'Medical Teacher' or title abbreviation: 'Med Teach' or the ISSN number: '1466-187X'. If you need to know the title abbreviation or the ISSN number of a journal, enter the full title and use the search tag 'Journal'. Then press ENTER or GO.	Searching a particular journal is less likely to be needed for your PBL learning issues search.

are commonly recommended as a resource in PBL rooms. *Dorland's Pocket Medical Dictionary, Merriam-Webster's* or the *Oxford Concise Medical Dictionary* are reasonably priced and are recommended to medical and healthcare students. Each student should have their own dictionary by the time they start their course.

TABLE 7.3 Medical dictionaries commonly used by medical and healthcare students

Dictionary	Publisher	Advantages
Dorland's Illustrated Medical Dictionary	Elsevier	Comprehensive, authoritative, illustrated resource for undergraduate and postgraduate students. Includes CD-ROM, PDA software and speller
Dorland's Pocket Medical Dictionary with CD-ROM	Saunders	Contains all essential terms needed by medical students Handy size
Melloni's Illustrated Medical Dictionary	The Parthenon Publishing Group	Comprehensive, authoritative, illustrated; for both undergraduate and postgraduate students
Melloni's Pocket Medical Dictionary Illustrated	The Parthenon Publishing Group	Illustrated Contains essential terms needed by medical students
Merriam-Webster's Medical Desk Dictionary	Merriam-Webster Incorporated	Contains essential terms needed by medical students
Mosby's Dictionary of Medicine, Nursing & Health Professions Australian and New Zealand edition	Elsevier	Fully illustrated Covers medical and allied healthcare needs
Oxford Concise Medical Dictionary	Oxford	Contains essential terms needed by medical students
Stedman's Medical Dictionary for the Health Professions and Nursing Australia/New Zealand edition	Lippincott Williams & Wilkins	Comprehensive, authoritative, illustrated; for both undergraduate and postgraduate students

Before using your dictionary read the notes on the use of the dictionary, the list of appendices and any other user information provided. Note that this information may be at the front or the back of the book and some of it may be on the inside covers.

EXERCISES

Here are four exercises to test your knowledge of your dictionary and your skills in using it as a research tool.

Exercise 1
Look for the sections that cover the following topics in your dictionary. Write down what the dictionary calls each section and the page numbers for each. Where do you find:
1 abbreviations used in the dictionary
2 frequently used stems
3 symbols, for example, the Greek alphabet, symbols used in pedigrees, symbols used in statistics
4 anatomical information, for example, bones, muscles, arteries, veins, nerves
5 the list of elements and temperature equivalents
6 help with pronunciation of a word
7 normal reference values
8 adult health assessment information
9 information on drugs and their pharmacological/toxicological effects
Some of the above are only dealt with in the large medical dictionaries. The contents pages will help you to discover other components of your dictionary.

Exercise 2
Practise finding individual terms as quickly as possible. Write down what you understand from the information provided by the dictionary for each of these terms.
1 Laparotomy
2 Jugular venous pressure
3 Caput medusae
4 Oximetry
5 Caudate lobe of the liver
6 Flexor carpi ulnaris
7 Spider angiomas
8 Basilar artery syndrome
9 Portal hypertension
10 Ataxia
11 Sinus rhythm

Exercise 3
What do these abbreviations stand for?
1 PUO
2 pH
3 LE
4 IVC
5 Li
6 Hb
7 HCV
8 AAFP
9 CEA
10 FSH

Exercise 4
Find the alternative Australian spelling for these words given in American spelling
1 Appendectomy
2 Cecum

3 Lipotropic
4 Anemia
5 Hemoglobin
6 Gynecomastia
7 Erythropoiesis
8 Eosinophil
9 Estrogen
10 Pediatrics

EFFECTIVE USE OF TEXTBOOKS
TEXTBOOKS: ONE OF THE MAIN RESOURCES

Textbooks, despite their limitations, are considered by course designers and students to be one of the main resources for learning. Advantages include:

- textbooks are written to student level
- most textbooks provide information in an educational framework using tools such as tables, flow charts and labelled images to summarise main points, application of knowledge or clinical cases and self-assessment questions at the end of each chapter
- some textbooks provide electronic multimedia resources with animation to facilitate understanding of difficult concepts
- textbooks are used by most lecturers to prepare their lectures and assessment questions
- textbooks cover the whole discipline. They are written to foster understanding of related topics
- textbooks are often written by several authors who are authorities in the areas addressed
- textbooks often include clinical examples, case scenarios and applications at the end of each chapter.

However, textbooks do have limitations which can be summarised as:

- Most textbooks are focused on one discipline and not integrated.
- Most textbooks are not written for PBL curricula.
- Textbooks are extensive and students need to learn how to use them.
- Epidemiological information in many textbooks can be limited or entirely absent. This information may be needed for PBL cases.
- Even medical textbooks do not teach students how to make differential diagnoses, structure the information needed, weigh the evidence for and against each hypothesis and develop a logical management approach that suits the patient.
- As most textbooks cover just one specialty they lack integrated discussion of mechanisms and pathogenesis.
- Many medical textbooks are deficient in the area of evidence-based medicine.

These limitations explain why we need resources other than textbooks and how important it is to use textbooks covering a number of disciplines as we prepare for our learning.

Let us say you are preparing your learning issues for a case on type 2 diabetes and hyperlipidaemia (increased serum cholesterol and triglycerides). One of the learning issues identified by your group is 'How are lipids transported in the body?'

Before you start let me ask you these questions:

- How will you start?

- Which textbooks will you choose? Why?
- What keywords will you choose in your search?
- Which textbook will you start with?
- How would you manage these two tasks?
  Having thought about these questions you can move on to the next exercise.

Exercise 5

1 In two or three textbooks read the chapters that cover type 2 diabetes and hyperlipidaemia.
2 Summarise the key information you have learnt. Make sure you include reference to how different lipids are transported.

IMPROVING LEARNING BY USING TEXTBOOKS

Step 1
- Think of what you know about the topic and write it down.
- Write down what might be covered in the textbook about this topic.
- Write down the keywords related to the topic.

Step 2
- Use the keywords you have identified to find the entries covering this topic in the book's index. Some books write the page numbers in **bold**, meaning that the majority of information regarding this topic can be found on those pages.
- Record what you find on the top right-hand corner of your notebook.
- In the contents pages look at the page numbers you found in the index and check which chapter(s) of the book they refer to. Are these chapters related to the topic you are researching?

Step 3
- Look at each chapter covering the topic.
- First look at the main headings in each chapter to get a better idea of what is covered. Then look at the subheadings.
- Look at the tables, flow charts and diagrams. Read their captions. Remember that tables, flow charts and diagrams summarise important elements of the chapter the author wants to bring to the reader's attention.

Step 4
- Go straight to the section of each chapter that seems most useful to you.
- Look at the first sentence of each paragraph: the topic covered in each paragraph is usually stated in the first sentence of the paragraph. This approach helps you find what the text is about.
- Ask yourself if you have found the answers for your questions. If so, record your findings.
- Write down what else you need to know.
- Continue this process in other sections and chapters.

Step 5
- Create your own material—diagrams, tables and flow charts—from the information you have searched.

- Your material should reflect your understanding of what you have read.

You may have chosen physiology, biochemistry and medical textbooks for your search. Any textbook from each of these disciplines will be fine. The keywords you decided to use for your search might have included:

- lipid transport
- cholesterol
- triglyceride
- lipoproteins
- hyperlipidaemia.

You may have looked at the medical textbook to get an overall picture about the topic then at the physiology and biochemistry texts for more information (see also Ch 5).

Exercise 6

- Summarise the key information you have learnt from the textbooks you selected.
- Would you like to use other resources as well? What would you choose? Why?

Here is a possible answer to the question, 'How are lipids transported in the body?'

- The major site for the synthesis of triacylglycerol (TG) and cholesterol is the liver. If there is excess of TG and cholesterol in excess of the liver's capacity, the liver mobilises these lipids into the blood, as low density lipoproteins (apo B-100 and apo E).
- TG in very low density lipoproteins and in chylomicrons is hydrolysed by lipases on the capillary surface, resulting in the production of intermediate-density lipoproteins.
- Low-density lipoprotein (LDL) carries cholesterol in blood and transports cholesterol to peripheral tissues.
- High-density lipoprotein (HDL) picks up cholesterol from dying cells and from cell membranes (called reversed cholesterol transport). These cholesterols are esterified by acyltransferase in HDL then returned by HDL to the liver.

Exercise 7

- What are the main problems in this summary?
- How would you improve this material?

PRESENTING INFORMATION FROM SEVERAL RESOURCES

- Focus on understanding.
- Use tables, flow charts and diagrams to construct the new information.
- Present difficult information clearly so you can remember it.
- Focus on key concepts and avoid redundant information.
- Think about clinical applications and uses.

See Appendix C for a better answer to the question in Exercise 6.

EFFECTIVE USE OF ONLINE RESOURCES

In the last two decades the internet has grown from a limited network for exchange of information between academics and government officials to a global communication system. This change has introduced major innovations in the practice of medicine and medical education. As a medical student you should be aware of current and possible future uses of *cybermedicine* (the process of applying the internet to medicine) and *medical informatics* (according to Wikipedia, 'the intersection of information science, computer science and health care') and during your undergraduate course you must develop the technical skills to work in this environment. The reasons for this include:

- The explosion in medical and health science information and research means all healthcare professionals need to keep learning and updating their knowledge after graduation.
- Patients regularly visit medical clinics with information obtained from the internet. Doctors should be prepared to answer their questions, explain whether the information provided was accurate or not and guide patients with appropriate information or educational websites. A number of doctors and healthcare professionals have developed their own websites and made links to local official medical and health societies. These can be used to guide patients to accurate sources of information.
- The move to computerised medical records. Medical history, investigation results, management and past treatment can easily be retrieved from these records by each member of the treating team.
- Increased access to *telemedicine*: the delivery of medicine at a distance by for instance, phone, satellite technology or video-conferencing when the provider and patient are located at a distance from each other.
- Use of telemedicine in conferences in medical and healthcare education.

WHAT MAKES A GOOD WEBSITE?

Many students find it difficult to decide which websites provide reliable information they can use for their learning. The criteria in Table 7.4 will help you identify educationally reliable websites to suit your needs.

See Appendix A for the URLs of educational websites on:
- clinical education resources
- drug information resources
- biomedical science resources
- clinical cases and pathology images
- gastrointestinal endoscopy
- medical dictionaries
- general resources.

USING COMPUTER-AIDED LEARNING (CAL) RESOURCES

There are many different names for computer-aided learning or computer-assisted learning (CAL): computer-assisted instruction (CAI), computer-based learning, and multimedia CD-ROMs. They all mean the same thing. Computer-aided learning resources in PBL:

- facilitate learning and understanding of difficult concepts (e.g. the use of three-dimensional liver structure and animations to explain the concept of double blood supply of the liver, sinusoids, bile flow, sinusoidal and canalicular domains of liver cells). These concepts may be difficult to understand from textbooks

TABLE 7.4 Criteria for evaluating educationally useful websites

Item	Assessment questions	Outcomes
1. Educational influence	Who published the website? Is it accredited by medical or scientific bodies? Do universities or other scientific bodies recommend its use? Is the website well organised and easy to search?	Make sure the publishers have supplied their name, address and copyright information. Websites recommended by universities and international scientific bodies are usually of good quality.
2. Purpose	What are the objectives of the website? What information does it provide? How detailed is the information provided? Do you feel the information provided corresponds with the website's objectives? Are there many advertisements?	Websites that focus on advertisements are less likely to be educationally useful.
3. Quality of information	Who wrote the content information? Are the authors expert in this area? Is the content edited and peer reviewed? Are there references at the end of each article? Are these references from peer-reviewed journals? Do the authors use a scientific approach in their writing? Is the content original? Is the content evaluated? Are there grammatical errors? Are the graphics and scientific images original?	Look for authors' credentials. Look for key editors, peer reviewers and if they are experts in the areas addressed. Referenced and peer-reviewed articles are educationally useful. Some websites provide detailed information about authors and a brief summary of their achievements and other publications.
4. Currency of information	When was the website last updated? Is consistency maintained in the website content? Are the references included in articles up-to-date? Are the links working? Is the information outdated?	A useful website is updated with current references.

- expand the concept of learning by doing. Most CAL programs are interactive: students complete activities to demonstrate their understanding of concepts discussed. These activities are followed by answers and feedback to improve the learner's skills

- allow students to add new skills and knowledge to what they have learnt and foster cognitive skills embedded in the curriculum. Some CAL programs are designed to match the PBL philosophy and consist of modules in a PBL case. By using these programs, learners improve their learning and problem-solving skills
- understand basic sciences and fine details related to PBL cases. Most PBL cases raise issues that require understanding of basic sciences. For example, a case on cystic fibrosis may require understanding of gas exchange, the genetic basis of cystic fibrosis and the molecular biology of the disease. Usually there is not enough time for discussing these details in PBL tutorials and learning these concepts through CAL programs is useful to students to complement their learning
- integrate basic and clinical sciences. Most CAL programs are integrated and foster application of knowledge learnt from basic sciences
- facilitate evidence-based learning. CAL programs covering evidence-based learning are very useful resources. They usually comprise modules that use clinical scenarios to encourage: (1) identification of problems, (2) generation of appropriate questions, (3) looking for supportive evidence to answer questions raised, (4) critical appraisal of evidence, and (5) reflection of learning acquired from the case. These CAL programs complement learning from PBL and clinical sessions.

WHAT MAKES A GOOD CAL RESOURCE?

Often students find it difficult to select a CAL program for their self-directed learning and cannot decide whether using such programs will help them or not. The following criteria should guide you. A useful CAL program:
- is designed for a PBL curriculum
- is interactive and provides students with the opportunity to complete tasks, work out problems, build models and answer questions
- integrates basic and clinical sciences
- is up-to-date, engaging and provides clear instructions to users
- provides feedback to foster learning
- has been evaluated by students and academics at different stages of its development
- enhances learner's cognitive skills
- uses animations, three-dimensional models and PBL cases to foster learning.

CONCLUSIONS

The challenges you can face in a PBL curriculum include finding the resources you need for your learning, developing the skills to use them effectively and building on your existing knowledge. This chapter has introduced you to the keys you need to master these challenges. Learning this information is never complete without putting each component into practice. Start with your subject guide, highlight key information you might need to refer to during the year, record in your reflective journal your plans for the semester, and orient yourself to different resources you might use. Learn how to search MEDLINE or other medical, biomedical and healthcare databases. Aim not only to find resources but also to master the skills of critically evaluating published papers and selecting appropriate resources to foster your learning. You need to assess the level of evidence provided and the different types of studies undertaken to assess evidence. Mastering these skills will enable you to distinguish between different views on a research issue and your own opinion and be able to justify your views. You also need to integrate knowledge and construct new information from several resources.

FURTHER READING
BOOKS

Cannon R, Newble D. A handbook for teachers in universities and colleges. 4th edn. London: Kogan Page; 1989.

Hartley J. Designing instructional text. 3rd edn. London: Kogan Page; 1994.

Knowles MS. Self-directed learning. A guide for learners and teachers. New York: Prentice Hall/Cambridge; 1975.

Newble DI, Cannon R. A handbook for medical teachers. 4th edn. Dordrecht, Netherlands: Kluwer Academic: 2001.

ARTICLES AND RESEARCH PAPERS

Azer SA. A multimedia CD-ROM tool to improve student understanding of bile salts and bilirubin metabolism: evaluation of its use in a medical hybrid PBL course. Adv Physiol Educ 2005; 29(1):40–50.

Bond CS, Fevyer D, Pitt C. Learning to use the Internet as a study tool: a review of available resources and exploration of students' priorities. Health Inform Libraries J 2006; 23(3):189–196.

Motschall E, Falck-Ytter Y. Searching the MEDLINE literature database through PubMed: a short guide. Onkologie 2005; 28(10):517–522.

Ruiz JG, Mintzer MJ, Leipzig RM. The impact of e-learning in medical education. Acad Med 2006; 81(3):207–212.

EVIDENCE-BASED LEARNING
Do we need dissection in an integrated problem-based learning medical course? Perceptions of first- and second-year students.

The introduction of a problem-based learning (PBL) curriculum at the School of Medicine of the University of Melbourne has necessitated a reduction in the number of lectures and limited the use of dissection in teaching anatomy. In the new curriculum, students learn the anatomy of different body systems using PBL tutorials, practical classes, pre-dissected specimens, computer-aided learning multimedia and a few dissection classes. The aims of this study are: (1) to assess the views of first- and second-year medical students on the importance of dissection in learning about anatomy, (2) to assess if students' views have been affected by demographic variables such as gender, academic background and being a local or an international student, and (3) to assess which educational tools helped them most in learning anatomy and whether dissection sessions have helped them in better understanding anatomy. METHODS: First- and second-year students enrolled in the medical course participated in this study. Students were asked to fill out a 5-point Likert scale questionnaire. Data was analysed using Mann-Whitney's U test, Wilcoxon's signed-ranks or the calculation of the Chi-square value. RESULTS: The response rates were 89% for both first- and second-year students. Compared to second-year students, first-year students perceived dissection to be important for deep understanding of anatomy (P < 0.001), making learning interesting (P < 0.001) and introducing them to emergency procedures (P < 0.001). Further, they preferred dissection over any other approach (P < 0.001). First-year students ranked dissection (44%), textbooks (23%), computer-aided learning (CAL), multimedia (10%), self-directed learning (6%) and lectures (5%) as the most valuable resources for learning anatomy, whereas second-year students found textbooks (38%), dissection (18%), pre-dissected specimens (11%), self-directed learning (9%), lectures (7%) and CAL programs (7%) as most useful. Neither of the groups showed a significant preference for pre-dissected specimens, CAL multimedia or lectures over dissection. CONCLUSIONS: Both first- and second-year students, regardless of their gender, academic background, or citizenship felt that the time devoted to dissection classes was not adequate. Students agreed that dissection deepened their understanding of anatomical structures, provided them with a three-dimensional perspective of structures and helped them recall what they learnt. Although their perception about the importance of dissection changed as they progressed in the course, good anatomy textbooks were perceived as an excellent resource for learning anatomy. Interestingly, innovations used in teaching anatomy, such as interactive multimedia resources, have not replaced students' perceptions about the importance of dissection.

For more information: http://www.springerlink.com/content/1279-8517/
Azer SA, Eizenberg N. Surg Radiol Anat 2007; 29(2):173–180. Epub 21 Feb, 2007.
    Adapted with permission from the publisher.

CHAPTER 8

Keys to foster study skills and learning attitude

> If we value independence, if we are disturbed by the growing conformity of knowledge, of values, of attitudes, which our present system induces, then we may wish to set up conditions of learning which make for uniqueness, for self-direction, and for self-initiated learning.
>
> **CARL ROGERS**

INTRODUCTION

Success in medicine or any other healthcare course is not based on how much information you learn during the course, or the quality of information you have acquired or how you can apply that information to real-life situations. Success is based on the competencies, skills and attitudes you have developed during your undergraduate years so you can cope with the challenges you will face when you graduate and practise as a healthcare professional.

Your attitude is the foundation of everything you do. It is the key for all processes controlling your destiny and professional life. Taking responsibility for your attitude very early in your course and preparing yourself for these changes should be your priority. Many researchers believe that a good attitude is not a product of genetics but can—with proper training—be acquired.

In medical and other healthcare courses there are a number of study skills you need to develop. You may already be aware of some of these from your high school years or a prior university course. These study skills and competencies include planning, time management, identifying priorities, organising your folders and discovering the power of self-motivation.

These skills are essential: you need not only to learn about them but also to master them so they become part of your learning attitude.

In this chapter I provide you with:

1 key information about a number of study skills that can enhance your learning attitude
2 examples and practical illustrations of these skills
3 tips to help you apply these skills in your learning and develop these competencies.

THINK PLANNING
WHAT IS THE PURPOSE OF PLANNING?

The purpose of planning is to:

- get a clear mental picture
- know what you ought to be doing on a day-to-day and on a long-term basis
- organise what you need to do
- keep track of work you have completed
- view the big picture as well as the fine details
- identify your priorities and plan how to manage your time.

Many students believe that planning is a waste of time, does not help them in their learning and is unnecessary. They believe that time spent planning doesn't produce any benefit; that many times what they plan for does not happen. Their plan may collapse because of casual work opportunities, unexpected visits by friends or feeling depressed. If your plan is not carefully designed, such opinions can be justified. If your plan is not designed to suit your needs, it is of no value.

Therefore your plan should be:

- realistic
- achievable
- reflective of your priorities
- suitable for your needs
- focused on your short-term and long-term objectives
- well organised
- thoroughly prepared
- not complex; easy to execute.

WHAT ARE THE KEY PRINCIPLES?

1 *Brainstorm what you need to do.* You may use a mind map or concept map in your approach. Brainstorming:
   — aims to generate new ideas on a specific issue
   — allows you to think freely
   — helps you establish patterns of thinking
   — provides you with the opportunity to examine a wide range of ideas
   — increases the richness of solutions and provides better decisions.
2 *Identify your working priorities.* When you have identified your learning priorities, you are able to design a useful plan for your work. Make a list of your priorities then rank them by giving each a score of 1 to 5 points, depending on how important it is to your learning needs. The questions in Box 8.1 will help you discover your learning priorities. See also the section below on 'First things first'.

BOX 8.1 How can I decide on my learning priorities?

What are my course objectives?
— What are my objectives for this week?
— What are the learning objectives I need to understand?
— What are the skills/competencies that I need to work on?
— What are the tasks I need to complete to achieve these skills/competencies?

How important are these tasks in improving my understanding and skills?
— How much is my time worth?
— How do I spend my time?
— How should I use my time?
— How much of my time do I spend on important learning tasks?
— How can I prioritise as well as do the other tasks I need to complete?

3 *Manage your time.* Planning, identifying your priorities and managing your time are key skills you will need not just for organising your learning needs during your undergraduate years but also when you graduate and practise medicine. Good time management is particularly important in the provision of patient care and the development of your life-long learning skills.

Review each item in your list and label them as important or not important and urgent or non-urgent.
— Group 'important and urgent' items together as Group 1.
— Group 'important and non-urgent' items together as Group 2.
— Group 'not important and urgent' items together as Group 3.
— Group 'not important and non-urgent' items together as Group 4.

Do not waste your time on items in Groups 3 and 4. Invest more time on items in Groups 1 and 2.

4 *Incorporate these tasks into an implementation plan.* A workable implementation plan allows you to:
— regulate your study time
— become organised
— set priorities
— achieve your goals on time
— not underestimate the time needed to complete a task.

5 *Be committed to what you plan.* The *Shorter Oxford English Dictionary* defines commitment as 'the action of committing oneself to a course of action; an engagement; an obligation; an act of committing oneself'. A committed person:
— keeps their plan working
— gives priority to tasks listed in their plan
— avoids interruptions or major changes to their plan
— works hard to compensate for any changes to their plan
— focuses on outcomes, not excuses
— feels they are 'in control'.

6 *Review and amend your plan as needed.*
— Tick tasks as you complete them.
— Keep your plan working.
— When necessary, make minor changes to your plan.

FIRST THINGS FIRST

The first step is to prioritise and focus on the competencies and skills tested at each stage of your course. This means you must you look ahead and prepare yourself for the next stage and see correlations in what you learn. Therefore you need to:
• study carefully the objectives of your course and those for each semester
• define the competencies and skills you need to develop at each stage
• identify priorities for your learning needs and tasks that can be grouped as 'learning priorities' (see Box 8.1).

Think also about these two key questions:
• How much of your time do you invest on your most important tasks?
• What system do you use to make your decisions?

Table 8.1 is a list of tasks and activities organised into four groups (1 to 4). They have been grouped on the basis of their importance and urgency.

TABLE 8.1 Tasks and activities organised on the basis of importance and urgency

Key questions	Group 1 Important and urgent	Group 2 Important and non-urgent	Group 3 Not important and urgent	Group 4 Not important and non-urgent
What examples can you supply for each group?	Deadlines (projects) Life crises Unexpected situations Traumatic changes Examinations Case presentations	Planning Self-development Improving learning skills Developing competencies Keeping fit Preparing for future challenges	Some emails Interruptions Unexpected visits from friends Leisure activities	Time-wasters Excessive TV watching, phoning, shopping, video gaming Unproductive activities
What do many students do with the items in each group?	Many students have a lot of things in this group to do. More items in this group means more exposure to stress and difficulties	Many students spend inadequate amounts of time on these tasks or delay working on them (e.g. leave writing assignment to 2 days before deadline)	Many students are trapped by activities in this section, spending a lot of time on them	Many students overdo these activities and waste their time
What should you do?	Move a number of tasks in this group to Group 2 to minimise the number of tasks in this group	Focus on this group to be well prepared for urgent and important tasks (e.g. examinations, deadlines etc)	Do not spend a lot of time on these activities	Be selective about these activities
What could you call each group?	'The place for few tasks'	'Developing and mastering competency'	'Activities to control'	'Time-wasting activities'

The lessons I would like to leave with you from Table 8.1 are:

1 Focus on items listed under Group 2 ('important and non-urgent') and invest more time on these tasks. The more you invest in these things, the more you will be able to achieve your dreams.

2 Avoid wasting your time on tasks you have included under Groups 3 and 4. Be selective.

3 Because some items in Group 1 can be moved to Group 2, you will minimise the number of 'important and urgent' tasks (Group 1) so you can perform at a high level with less stress.

MANAGE YOUR TIME

You may think that good time management is the ability to complete more tasks faster. Although this definition appears logical, attractive and of some use, the reality is that increasing your speed may not be the best solution and may actually make things more difficult. For example, it might reinforce superficial learning and change your focus from quality achievement to quantity achievement. Over time, you may become dependent on an attitude of urgency, being overly zealous about getting more things done in less time.

Managing your time well will provide you with the opportunity to:

• develop your competencies and skills in areas of need
• enjoy the work you are doing
• achieve your goals with minimal stress (optimise your effort)
• become more focused on important and non-urgent things (activities that will give you the greatest return)
• become more confident in your work
• progress in your work
• be in control of what you are doing
• become aware of the value of time and avoid time wasting
• learn how to use your time effectively.

Why do people feel both overworked and unproductive?

• They have not learnt how to organise themselves.
• They do not process their work.
• They have not learnt how to plan their work and use their time effectively.
• They focus on 'not important and non-urgent' things.

Read the time management skills questionnaire in Box 8.2 and choose your answer for each question.

TIME MANAGEMENT TIPS

Have any of these thoughts ever crossed your mind? 'I am doing my best but I do not feel that I am achieving or progressing in my learning' 'How can I maximise my achievements?' 'Is there anything I need to change?' 'What options do I have?' 'I feel time flies' 'I cannot find time to study' 'I am not in control'.

You might at times feel overwhelmed with similar thoughts. You may become occupied and feel challenged and disempowered. Most students who share such thoughts are in fact challenged by poor time management skills.

Developing time management skills is a long journey that you should start early in your course. Reading these tips is the beginning but you need to apply them as you journey.

BOX 8.2 Test your time management skills				
Do you construct a daily time plan?				
(1) Never	(2) Seldom	(3) Sometimes	(4) Often	(5) Always
Do you set specific goals for each study session?				
(1) Never	(2) Seldom	(3) Sometimes	(4) Often	(5) Always
Do you put your plans into action?				
(1) Never	(2) Seldom	(3) Sometimes	(4) Often	(5) Always
How often does your time plan become non-workable?				
(1) Never	(2) Seldom	(3) Sometimes	(4) Often	(5) Always
Do you look at what is preventing you from achieving your goals?				
(1) Never	(2) Seldom	(3) Sometimes	(4) Often	(5) Always

Calculate your scores for each question and find the significance of your total score:
5–10: Lacking planning skills
11–15: Low planning skills
16–20: Average planning skills
21–25: High planning skills

1 Determine how you plan to spend a typical day.
   — What activities do you need to accomplish?
   — How many hours will you allocate for each task?
   — What are your objectives?
2 Make priorities.
   — What are the tasks you need to complete which can be classified as 'important and non-urgent'?
   — Will these tasks give you the maximum return?
   — What skills and competencies do you need to develop?
   — What will you lose if you do not start working on these issues?
3 Avoid time-wasters.
   — What are your time-wasters? List them.
   — How will you deal with or avoid your time-wasters?
   — Credit yourself each time you succeed in avoiding time-wasters.
4 Set your own deadlines.
   • Your own deadlines should be 3–4 days earlier than what has been set.
   • Use the remaining time in revision and improving the quality of your work.
5 Develop the habit of time management (Box 8.3). Developing a new habit takes time, a lot of work and commitment. It does not develop overnight. The important thing is to believe in your abilities and focus on developing good habits. The skill of time management is vital for you, not only during your undergraduate years but also after graduation when you practise medicine. The following actions may be of use:
• record your daily time management approach
• always think about the benefits of time management
• read books about time management
• identify obstacles that affect your time management plans
• replace bad habits with good ones. See Table 8.2 for a few examples. In your

BOX 8.3 Developing the habit of time management will:

— reduce avoidance and delaying what you should do
— reduce anxiety
— give you enough time to complete tasks effectively
— promote production
— save time.

TABLE 8.2 Replace bad habits with good ones

Bad habit	Change to
'I rushed to do my assignment at the last minute … I was really stressed'	'By planning what I need to do and organising my time, I am able to manage my work with minimal stress'
'I spent a lot of time searching for a paper … I cannot remember where I placed it'	'By organising my paper and electronic folders, I can easily find any document I need and save a lot of time'
'I am behind in my studies'	'By organising my time, I feel in control'
'I always come late to the PBL tutorials and find it difficult to join in the discussion …'	'By coming on time to tutorials, I am more able to join in the discussion'
'I missed yesterday's lecture … I thought we did not have a lecture at 3 pm'	'By reviewing my schedule in the morning, I can prepare myself for each session'

reflective journal you might add more items that reflect your needs. For each item, write down the good habits you will develop instead.
6 Plan to make the best out of your time.
   — Be clear about what you want to achieve.
   — Be passionate about your work and achievements.
   — Be creative in the use of your time.
   — Create a 'do it' list.
   — Develop a daily/weekly planner.
   — Develop a long-term planner.
7 Overcome procrastination. (Procrastination means putting off things that you should be focusing on right now.)
   — What are the causes of your procrastination?
   — How can procrastination affect your learning progress?
   — What can you do to avoid procrastination?

ORGANISE YOUR COMPUTER FOLDERS

Throughout your course, digital documents will be a vital component of your folders. Digital documents can include email, web pages, PowerPoints, lecture notes, learning issues, study summaries, electronic reflective journals and review papers. As it is easy to create and receive digital documents, they tend to proliferate more than paper documents. While storage of digital documents is relatively easy and does not take space in your room, finding these documents is sometimes time consuming and difficult. Therefore, it is essential to organise your digital documents. Organisation will allow you to:

- find any document you need
- keep you 'in control'
- manage your learning without wasting your time.
    Use the following tips to organise your electronic folders and your documents.

1 Create a 'My Document' folder (if not already on your C: drive). Create three subject folders (directories) in My Document. Give them the following titles, '1Current', '2References', '3Archives'. By putting the number '1' next to the name that file will be placed at the top of the 'My Document' tree; the file with number '2' next to the name will be placed second in the 'My Document' tree and so on.

2 Create subfolders, for example, 'Semester 1' folder and 'Semester 2' folder, if you have two semesters per year. Under each semester folder, create subfolders, one folder for each week of the semester, you may call them, 'Week1', 'Week2', 'Week3', etc. Or you could create a subfolder for 'Weeks 1 to 5', a second subfolder for 'Weeks 6 to 10' and a third subfolder for 'Weeks 11 to 15'. This will depend on your exact needs and the structure of your course.

3 Under the '1Current' folder and using, for example, 'Week1' subfolder of Semester 1, you might place the following documents:
    — problem-based learning (PBL) issues, diagrams and group discussion
    — lecture notes
    — your own summaries and study notes
    — introduction to clinical medicine study paper
    — diagrams, flow charts, mechanisms, etc.

4 Under the '2References' folder and using, for example, 'Week1' subfolder of semester 1, you might place the following documents:
    — PowerPoints
    — journal articles
    — review papers
    — other resources.

5 Under the '3Archives' folder and using, for example, 'Week 1' subfolder of Semester 1 of last year, you might place all the documents you had related to this week. This will allow you to move documents to the archive folders at the end of the year.

6 Always back up all documents on your external hard drive.

DISCOVER THE POWER OF SELF-MOTIVATION

Self-empowerment and self-motivation are powerful sources for your success, particularly when you know how to use them for a specific purpose. A number of physiological and psychological functions control your self-motivation. These functions are affected by a number of factors including:

- internal messages you keep sending yourself
- previous experiences and current challenges
- what you think about yourself and the people around you
- your dreams
- your ability to deal with challenges
- what you see as priorities
- how you handle stress
- cultural beliefs.

Despite these factors, self-motivation can be learnt and developed if you keep working on developing this skill. The keys for self-motivation can be summarised as:

→ KEY 1 VISUALISE OUTCOMES

A picture or a mental picture of what you want to end with is more empowering than words. You know this from your own experience. A few years ago, I met a student who dreamed of becoming a medical student at the University of Melbourne. She told me that deep inside she wanted her dream to come true. She kept thinking about this wonderful desire and visualised herself as a student in the course. To reinforce her desire she collected pictures of medical students, stethoscopes and the university. She placed these photos in her room over her bed. She believes that this technique of daily visualisation of her dreams helped her achieve her goals.

The more you visualise what you want to achieve, the easier it will be to attain. Many professional athletes spend a considerable amount of time on their mental training. They use visualisation to see themselves progress through every step of their training. At cellular and molecular levels, there is evidence that the practice of visualisation enhances neuromuscular signals, neurochemical communication and neuromuscular coordination, leading to successful performance in actual events.

Why is visualisation useful in building your self-motivation?
- It keeps you thinking about your goals and final outcomes.
- It allows you to look at your goals from many different viewpoints.
- It gives you the clarity to act on things that are the most important to your project.
- The mental images you create make you believe you can reach your goals.
- It keeps reminding you of your priorities.
- Gradually, these mental images will create feelings of achievement, success and a desire for more success.

→ KEY 2 AFFIRM YOUR SUCCESS

An affirmation is a set of words and messages that can improve your confidence and be a positive element in your mind. It can involve stating something you believe to be true even when in current circumstances it appears to be contradicted. An affirmation contains the elements of your self-motivation, survival dynamics, life goals, and personal achievements. As you repeat these statements, you become self-motivated. These words should be in the present tense, simple, active and carry positive messages.

Examples of affirmations you can use:
'I am enjoying my studies'
'I feel complete confidence in my skills and abilities'
'I know I can achieve anything I set my mind to'
'I know I can do anything I plan to do to improve my learning'
'I know that nothing is impossible for me'
'I feel confident'
'I am awesome'
'I possess dreams and the determination to accomplish my goals'
'Deep inside me, I believe in myself and my abilities'

'I was born for success'

'I am organised'

'I am capable of planning and managing my life'

If you say powerful statements like these for 5 minutes at a time each day, your mindset will be energised and your confidence in yourself and your abilities will be dramatically increased. Write the statements in your reflective journal.

Many successful people believe that life is 10 per cent what happens to us and 90 per cent how we respond to it. Your response is more important than your past, your education, your fame or what other people think of you or say about you.

Why is an affirmation of your success useful?

- It enables you to believe in yourself.
- It gives you a willingness to achieve.
- It gives you a positive state of mind.
- It makes the present moment your happiest.
- It empowers you as you face challenges.
- It keeps you 'in control'.

→ KEY 3 REWARD YOURSELF

We all feel better when we are rewarded for doing a task. The reward means that we are doing well, that our achievement is important to others. Such feelings motivate us to continue working and make us feel happy about ourselves. Unfortunately there are many situations on a daily basis where there is no one around to give you a reward or say things such as 'Good job', 'That is excellent', 'Great work', 'Your input was very useful to the group', or 'Keep up the good work'. And not all teachers reward their students or are available to support and acknowledge good work. If this is the case, you may at times feel discouraged or want somebody to say encouraging words that will motivate you. Rewarding yourself is very useful in such situations.

→ KEY 4 KEEP ENGAGED

One of the meanings of the word 'engage' in the *Macquarie Dictionary* is 'drop down of the fetus' head into the mother's pelvis in preparation for birth'. Self-motivation is not just about visualisation, affirmation and rewarding yourself, it is also about moving ahead and engaging as if you have realised your goals. This process is essential in self-motivation. Take every possible action to advance your dreams. See the significance of your work and keep moving towards your goal. Do not wait: be proactive and dynamic.

→ KEY 5 ENERGISE YOURSELF

Your body language says a lot about your thoughts. You can use your body to change your mental state and how you feel about yourself. For example, sit straight, head high and change your breathing to a deep, slow abdominal breathing. Change your facial expression; smile to become more positive and determined. By making these physical changes, even if you feel down, you will gradually be able to: (1) energise your muscles to control your emotions, and (2) deal with upsetting situations. This skill needs a lot of practice but gradually you will be able to control your feelings and energise yourself even in difficult situations.

→ KEY 6 BE PERSISTENT

Persistence enhances your self-motivation and empowers you to focus on your dreams. Your self-motivation empowers your persistence and determination and hence, your success. This mutual interaction between persistence and self-motivation is one of the key elements for success. If you read the biographies of successful people you will find that most of them discovered this relationship and invested a lot of their time in using this interaction to overcome obstacles and failures. For example, Thomas Edison, inventor of the light bulb, the Wright brothers, inventors of the first aeroplane and Marconi, inventor of the wireless, all dreamed of their inventions and after hundreds, even thousands of trials and failures, succeeded in making their dreams a reality.

IMPROVE YOUR CONCENTRATION

HOW CAN YOU INCREASE LEARNING CONCENTRATION?

- Plan what you want to do.
- Take a shower before starting your study.
- Organise your desk and use a comfortable chair.
- Avoid distractors (see Box 8.4).
- Allocate enough time for each task you do.
- Become engaged: search for answers, think laterally, reflect on what you have learnt, use several resources, identify new questions, think about the clinical applications of knowledge gained from basic sciences, think about the use of information to solve a similar problem.
- Take notice of what you have learnt, read loud and use analogies when needed.
- Use diagrams or construct simple models to increase your understanding.
- Train yourself to do one thing at a time.
- Take short breaks every 50–90 minutes.
- Reward yourself when you complete a task.
- Visualise your success and your achievements.

HOW TO MINIMISE TIME WASTED BY DISTRACTORS

- Choose a place for your study that allows you to be away from your distractors. For example, a quiet place in the library may be better than your home if other people, your pet or television are the main sources of your distraction.
- Set aside periods for planning, covering short-term and long-term needs.
- Ask yourself if there are some aspects of study that you are not doing as well as you should.
- Plan your time off and use it as a reward after doing work. This will minimise distraction and interruption of your study.
- Count the hours you spent on distractors last week. List the items that can be avoided or minimised. Think about modifying your schedule to accommodate these changes. Be realistic in your planning.
- Turn your phone off or put it on silent.

BOX 8.4 What are your distractors?

Everyone should be aware of their distractors. These may be:
— video games
— watching television
— excessive use of mobile phones
— going out for coffee
— emails
— demanding friends
— pets
— going out, parties
— magazines
— shopping
— excessive casual/part-time work.
　　Identify your main distractors from this list and add any that apply to you that are not listed here. Rank each distractor as +++, ++, or + depending on the time you spend on each, with +++ meaning 4–5 hours per day, ++ meaning 2–3 hours per day and + meaning 1 hour per day. Calculate the number of hours you waste on a daily basis. Think about strategies you might use to minimise this time wasting.

MONITOR YOUR PROGRESS

Why is it important to monitor your progress?
- Self-monitoring provides you with a true perspective.
- Self-monitoring helps you clarify the big picture.
- Self-monitoring enables you to turn a good experience into a valuable experience you can gain from.
- Self-monitoring helps you identify deficiencies in your competencies.

HOW CAN YOU MONITOR YOUR PROGRESS?

- Use a reflective journal to record your learning experiences.
- Use your critical thinking skills to assess your achievements.
- Compare your achievements with the competencies and skills identified by the faculty for each stage of the course.
- Study your tutor's report and their feedback to you.
- Write out your action plan to enhance your skills in areas of need.
- Evaluate your progress as you implement your plan.

　　The seven characteristics of people who monitor their progress are that they:
1 have strong self-belief
2 focus on quality improvement and personal development
3 are persistent
4 improve their skills in a progressive way over time
5 focus on solutions
6 are willing to receive feedback
7 take action to improve their attitude.

ASK FOR HELP

Asking for help:
- allows you to discuss issues that worry you
- allows you to receive information and find answers to your questions
- helps you manage difficult situations
- provides you with new insights and new options
- helps you to make decisions, particularly about serious issues
- provides you with supportive resources
- provides you with feedback and ways to improve your performance and learning strategies.

WHO DO YOU ASK FOR HELP?

Depending on what is required and the areas you need help in, you might choose to ask for help from:
- members of the 'buddy program'
- your PBL tutor
- the subject guide and faculty website
- semester coordinator
- academic mentor
- members of your PBL group
- university counsellor
- student support program.

USE FEEDBACK TO IMPROVE YOUR SKILLS

Feedback is important to you. It gives you insight into your performance, areas of strength and areas that need development. It can alert you to the need to make or change priorities, and how to do that. Look for feedback from your tutor and work out how to get the most from it.

Successful students:
- regard feedback as a valuable opportunity
- do not get defensive when feedback is critical
- are proactive and ask their mentors/tutors to give them feedback
- use feedback to improve their performance
- do not take critical feedback personally: they prefer to thank their tutors for feedback, whether it is positive or negative.

HOW TO PREPARE FOR A FEEDBACK SESSION

- Remember that the aim of feedback is to build you up. Without feedback there would be no champions. Therefore, feedback is not for giving you bad news.
- Be willing to listen to your tutor and discuss questions they ask you during the interview.
- If you do not agree with your tutor, do not try to defend your position or argue. It is better to listen and think about the points they raise.
- Be clear in what you say. Always tell the truth and use the session as an opportunity to build trust and rapport with your tutor.
- Focus on values and show interest in what is discussed in the session.

- Ask your tutor how they can help you and who else might be of use.
- Ask your tutor if they think you need to meet again and what tasks you could work on between meetings.

QUESTIONS ASKED DURING FEEDBACK

Your tutor will make a time to see each student in the group individually. The interview sessions are usually held in week 4 or 5 of the semester. Your tutor may explain to the group the aims of the session: to see how you are going and to discuss areas you might need to improve. Sessions are usually about 20–25 minutes long and held in a PBL room or your tutor's room. To keep the process standardised most faculties have developed criteria for tutor assessment. You should be aware of the criteria used and understand its content. You may find a copy in your subject guide or on the faculty website.

Questions that might be raised by a tutor include:
- How do you feel you are going?
- How do you feel about your input to the group?
- What are the areas you feel you are excelling in?
- What do you think about our group?
- What are the areas you think you need to work on?
- Is there anything stopping you?
- How could we work together on this issue?
- Do you have any suggestions?
- What are the things you will work on till we see each other next?
- Should I talk on your behalf to our support team?
- If yes, what would you like me to say?

LEARN TO MANAGE STRESS

Stress is a mental or physical tension, strain or pressure. It fatigues people and makes them less productive. An excellent definition of stress is provided by Doc Childre and Howard Martin in their book *The HeartMath Solution*:

> Stress is the body and mind's response to any pressure that disrupts their normal balance. It occurs when our perceptions of events don't meet our expectations and we don't manage our reaction to the disappointment. Stress—that unmanaged reaction—expresses itself as resistance, tension, strain, or frustration, throwing off our physiological and psychological equilibrium and keeping us out of sync. If our equilibrium is disturbed for long, the stress becomes disabling. We fade from overload, feel emotionally shut down, and eventually get sick.

Medical and other healthcare students are vulnerable to stress for a number of reasons: (1) the nature of the curriculum and course design, (2) countless hours of study, (3) strenuous examinations, (4) financial issues for some students, and (5) the constant demand to perform to the standards of the course. For this reason most medical and healthcare schools provide information and training sessions to first-year medical students during the first few weeks and again at mid-semester about learning skills and dealing with stress. Box 8.5 summarises examples of topics that might be included in such programs.

> **BOX 8.5** Examples of topics discussed in orientation and students' wellbeing programs
> — stress management skills, relaxation techniques and time management skills
> — student wellbeing skills, physical and psychological health
> — vulnerability of medical and healthcare students to stress and substance abuse
> — planning and organisational skills
> — support systems available to students including peer support system.

WHAT ARE THE KEY PRINCIPLES OF STRESS?

Principle 1: Not all stress is bad. If you know how to manage your stress you can use it to help you succeed. For example, the stress associated with examinations could empower you to focus on what you need to do, concentrate your thoughts, use your time effectively and review the whole subject before the examination.

Principle 2: People differ in their reaction to stress. What one person considers stressful, another may not find stressful at all. There are many reasons for these differences:

— personality: people with type A personalities are described as being impatient, extremely competitive, always in a hurry, chronically angry, hard workers, ambitious and easily irritated by delays and interruptions. They are more susceptible to stress
— upbringing and cultural background
— moving to a new environment; language and cultural barriers
— past experiences, skills, attitude and training to deal with stressful situations
— environmental and circumstantial factors such as lack of support, financial problems, workload, family problems
— health problems
— low self-esteem and lack of confidence
— poor interpersonal skills.

Principle 3: Not all stress is equal. Certain emotional states are more damaging than others. The emotions that are most damaging are depression, anger, worry, frustration, anxiety, grief, guilt and rage.

Principle 4: Preventive strategies will help you be less vulnerable to stress, for example, prior training on how to manage stress and knowledge about the course structure and the skills you needs to develop. Also helpful are prior knowledge and practice of planning, organisation, time management and self-motivation skills.

Principle 5: Seek help. Do not ignore your stress or pretend you are fine. Continuous stress can create health problems and should be managed at an early stage.

BODY CHANGES IN STRESS

When we become stressed, a number of physiological and biochemical changes occur in our body and the signs that result from these changes may be: (1) reduced concentration, (2) loss of self esteem, (3) hesitation, (4) impaired judgement, (5) sleep disturbance, (6) depression, and (7) lack of energy and enthusiasm. Stress can even result in suicide.

Most of our body systems are troubled by stress particularly when it continues for some time. These troubles can be summarised as follows:

Cardiovascular problems:
— Hypertension
— Palpitation
— Dizziness and lightheadedness

Respiratory problems:
— Shortness of breath
— Hyperventilation
— Bronchospasm
— Chronic recurrent colds, sore throats, ear infection, sinus infection
— Recurrent bronchitis
— Activation of asthma

Musculoskeletal problems:
— Chronic back pain
— Fibromyalgia
— Tendonitis
— Chronic pain syndrome
— Tremors of hands

Headaches:
— Tension headaches
— Migraine headaches

Genitourinary problems:
— Loss of sex drive
— Frequent urination
— Chronic yeast infection

Gastrointestinal problems:
— Gastroesophageal reflux
— Heartburn
— Indigestion
— Irritable bowel syndrome

Skin conditions:
— Eczema
— Acne
— Activation of psoriasis
— Skin rash

Immune related problems and allergies:
— Chronic and recurrent infections
— Allergic rhinitis
— Food allergies

SOURCES OF STRESS FOR STUDENTS

Few studies have examined medical and healthcare students' stress associated with PBL. If students are school leavers or have completed other courses at university they may find PBL quite daunting. This, together with the stressors involved in adapting to changes such as moving from another country to study and using English in the course when students are from a non-English-speaking background, may add to pressure during initial exposure to PBL.

Other sources of stress associated with PBL may include:

- In PBL, students are expected to determine their own learning objectives, decide on the appropriate resources they need to research for information and decide when their learning is adequate.
- In PBL, students need to work collaboratively in small groups, discuss cases and learn from other members in the group. This may differ from their expectations because they were trained to compete and were accepted into the course on the basis of their competition with many other applicants.
- In small-group learning, students need to demonstrate effective communication and interpersonal skills such as debating, listening, teamwork and collaboration. Most students who are trained in a traditional teaching system do not possess these skills and may be stressed by the demands of their new course.
- Some students in PBL feel that they have a responsibility to keep their group functioning despite stress caused by conflict in the group or by the dominance of one or two members or by poor facilitation by their tutor. This may add to their stress, particularly when they do not know how to handle such situations.
- In addition to these stressors, students in PBL tutorials need to demonstrate a number of cognitive skills such as generation of hypotheses, constructing mechanisms, collecting new information, making decisions, verifying evidence for and against each hypothesis and interpreting clinical and laboratory investigations. Some of the students who come from a traditional course may find learning in PBL tutorials stressful and demanding.

Two research papers have addressed medical and physiotherapy students' stress associated with PBL. The first paper is by Gisele Mouret, a surgical resident from Royal North Shore Hospital in Sydney: 'Stress in a graduate medical degree' and the second paper is by Patricia Solomon and Elspeth Finch from McMaster University in Canada: 'A qualitative study identifying stressors associated with adapting to problem-based learning'. The factors causing stress in first-year medical students, as outlined in Mouret's paper, are shown in Figure 8.1.

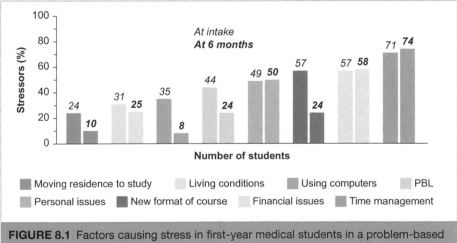

FIGURE 8.1 Factors causing stress in first-year medical students in a problem-based graduate entry course.

The figure was created from data provided by Mouret GML. Med J Aust 2002; 177: S10–S11. Adapted with permission from the publisher.

The data from Mouret's paper demonstrate that in a graduate medical PBL course, first-year students find the course stressful; the main factors being related to time management and financial issues. However, stress associated with PBL dropped from about 44 per cent at the start of the course to 24 per cent 6 months later. Similarly, stress related to the use of computers dropped from 35–8 per cent and stress related to the format of the course dropped from 57–24 per cent. However, time management, financial issues and personal issues remained as sources of their stress even 6 months after commencing the course. For physiotherapy students, stressors related to adapting to PBL are summarised in Table 8.3.

TABLE 8.3 Factors causing stress in first-year physiotherapy students (total number = 165)	
Stressor	**Number (percentage)**
Uncertainty of breadth and depth of knowledge required	26 (65.0)
Time pressures	26 (65.0)
Lack of confidence to adapt to PBL	19 (47.5)
Misunderstanding of PBL and faculty roles	17 (42.5)
Unrealistic expectations of self	15 (37.5)
Group learning	14 (35.0)
Workload	13 (32.5)
Search stress	13 (32.5)
Process evaluation	11 (27.5)
Group panic	11 (27.5)

Adapted from Solomon P, Finch E. Teach Learn Med 1998; 10(2):58–64

From the results given in these two papers we can draw the following conclusions:
- There are similarities in the stressors associated with PBL regardless of the type of course.
- Other sources of stress such as time management, financial issues, personal issues and new format of the course can add to stress associated with PBL.
- The 'buddy program' may help to decrease stress levels.

WHAT SHOULD YOU DO TO MANAGE YOUR STRESS?

Use the tips discussed below to manage your stress.
1 Do not take yourself too seriously.
2 Be prepared for difficult situations. During your undergraduate years and after graduation you will face a number of challenges and stressful situations. By being prepared to handle stress, you will be more able to handle difficult situations with minimal stress.
3 Avoid the blame game. The blame game perpetuates bitterness and resentment. Continually ruminating about past injustices will only deepen these feelings. The common statements of a bitter person are:
      'I do not deserve this'
      'Why me?'
      'Nobody cares about what happens to me'
      'Why am I singled out?'

'This is unfair'

'I know they do not like me'

Such statements will cripple you and make you feel upset. Stop grievances from developing by remaining positive.

4 Replace negative thoughts with positive and encouraging ones. Negative thoughts that encourage self-doubt are not useful. For example, 'I don't know if I can really complete this task. It is more complicated than I thought'. Your reaction to a situation will make a big difference. See the good things in what happens. Do not see yourself as powerless. Use the power of positive thinking by saying, for example:

'This time things were not okay, but most of the time, things go well'

'I have failed in this situation, but it is not the end of the world. In fact, I have enjoyed my work and this situation has given me new ideas'

'I have made a mistake, but there are a number of good things I can do'

5 Reflect and relax. There are a number of techniques to help you to relax:

— deep abdominal breathing

— yoga

— meditation and prayers

— exercise

— aerobic exercise

— massage.

6 Remember laughter is a good medicine.

7 Seek help. Do not be afraid to seek help if your stress continues for more than 2 weeks or you become unable to manage your usual workload. There are a number of people in your faculty who can help you:

— your academic mentor

— university counselling service

— your general practitioner

— student wellbeing and support group on your campus

— peer support systems—available for junior students. In this system first-year students are paired with second- or third-year students on a one-to-one basis or in a group.

CONCLUSIONS

This chapter gives you a number of strategies to foster your study skills including planning for success, defining priorities and managing time effectively, organising computer folders, discovering the power of self-motivation, improving your concentration, monitoring your progress, using feedback and managing your stress. I strongly advise you to start putting these learning strategies into practice and use your reflective journal to critically analyse your achievements. Try to avoid being distracted and stopping work on these skills. Give them priority when you start your course: for the first few weeks invest more of your time on using and testing these skills than on the lectures, tutorials and content. Once you have mastered them, you will find yourself moving rapidly and with confidence across any material you want to learn. You will appreciate every moment you spent organising yourself and developing these skills, particularly when you need to prepare for examinations, develop new skills or competencies and improve your learning attitude. Start working on these skills today.

EVIDENCE-BASED LEARNING
Student-led stress management program for first-year medical students

The medical education community has emphasized repeatedly the importance of teaching stress management and self-care skills to medical students. However, descriptions and evaluations of intervention programs are infrequent. This paper describes a student-led stress management program for first-year medical students and summarises program evaluation data from the participants. Method: The Stress Management Program is a voluntary activity that involves small groups of first-year medical students meeting with second-year student coleaders. At the beginning of the fall semester, each group meets one hr per week for seven consecutive weeks. Two psychologist faculty members serve as program coordinators. The evaluation of the program showed that the mean annual participation rate for first-year students was 94% over 16 years. Program evaluation results are strongly positive. The authors concluded that based on longevity of the program, high participation, and positive student feedback, the program has been successful.'

Redwood SK, Pollak MH. Teach Learn Med 2007, 19(1):42–46. Adapted with permission from the publisher.
For more information: http://www.siumed.edu/tlm/

FURTHER READING
BOOKS

Childre DL, Martin H. The HeartMath solution: The Institute of HeartMath's revolutionary program for engaging the power of the heart's intelligence. New York: HarperCollins; 1999.

Hettich PI. Learning skills for college and career. 2nd edn. Pacific Grove: Brooks/Cole, 1998.

Nelson AP, Gilbert S. Harvard medical school guide to achieving optimal memory. Harvard Medical School Guides. New York: McGraw-Hill; 2005.

Schunk DH, Zimmerman BJ. Self-regulated learning: From teaching to self-reflective practice. New York: The Guilford Press; 1998.

ARTICLES AND RESEARCH PAPERS

Frank E, Carrera JS, Stratton T, et al. Experiences of belittlement and harassment and their correlates among medical students in the United States: longitudinal survey. BMJ 2006; 333(7570):682.

Finkelstein C, Brownstein A, Scott C, et al. Anxiety and stress reduction in medical education: an intervention. Med Educ 2007; 41(3): 258–264.

Misch DA. Andragogy and medical education: are medical students internally motivated to learn? Adv Health Sci Educ Theory Prac 2002; 7(2):153–160.

Mouret GML. Stress in a graduate medical degree. Med J Aust 2002; 177:S10–S11.

Redwood SK, Pollak MH. Student-led stress management program for first-year medical students. Teach Learn Med 2007, 19(1):42–46.

Saipanish R. Stress among medical students in a Thai medical school. Med Teach 2003; 25(5):502–506.

Solomon P, Finch E. A qualitative study identifying stressors associated with adapting to problem-based learning. Teach Learn Med 1998; 10(2):58–64.

The student and the junior doctor in distress—"Our duty of care". Proceedings of a conference of the Confederation of Postgraduate Medical Education Councils 19–20 July 2001. Med J Aust 2002; 177(1 Suppl):S1–S32.

CHAPTER 9

Portfolios and reflective journals

> Without reflection, we go blindly on our way, creating more unintended consequences, and failing to achieve anything useful.
>
> **MARGARET J WHEATLEY**

INTRODUCTION

Examinations are not the only means of assessing students' competencies, skills and knowledge. In recent years medical, nursing and other schools have introduced portfolios and reflective journals as learning and assessment tools. The aim is not to replace examinations but to add new tools that can provide particular perspectives about students' learning and their progress. The information gained is different from that obtained from examinations: it provides students and faculties with a number of useful outcomes, for example, the ability to deal with challenges, how to plan solutions and how learning experiences enhance skills.

A *portfolio* is a collection of work that represents a student's learning, progress and achievement over time. Portfolios can be used to (1) capture evidence of a learner's competency and personal and professional growth, (2) assess development of critical thinking and written reflections, and (3) provide learners with the opportunity to evaluate their behaviour and practices. For example, students can reflect on their personal and professional development by looking at the entries that mark out their experiences and how these demonstrate the skills they have developed.

As portfolios are a new concept with several variations in their use, schools usually introduce students gradually to them and to reflective journals—which are often a component of the portfolios. Some conduct workshops at different stages of the semester to ensure that students have grasped the concepts behind portfolios and are able to construct their own reflective journals effectively. In this chapter I (1) introduce you to the structure, design, use and development of portfolios, (2) provide you with ideas and tips to get the best from your reflective journals, and (3) show you examples and practical applications of reflective journals in a problem-based learning (PBL) curriculum.

WHAT IS A PORTFOLIO?

The *Shorter Oxford English Dictionary* defines a portfolio as 'a case, in the form of a large book-cover, for holding loose sheets of paper, drawings, maps, music, etc'. Portfolios are used in undergraduate and postgraduate courses such as architecture, fine arts, photography, nursing, medicine and engineering to assess students' learning. They help students capture learning from daily experiences. Consider the following points as we discuss the definition of a portfolio:

- There are variations in the concept and use of portfolios. In fact, there are over nine different types of portfolios reported in the literature and each school has its own structure and requirements. 'Assessment portfolios' document students' learning on specific learning outcomes, 'skills area portfolios' demonstrate acquired skills in specific areas such as PBL and 'reflective portfolios' focus on critical reflection, learning experiences and provision of supportive evidence from learning.
- Portfolios may be organised by the user in different ways. However, each school usually provides its students with guidelines and instructions about portfolio organisation and scope. This ensures standardisation of marking and helps students to better design their portfolios.
- A reflective portfolio, also known as a *reflective journal*, encourages students to focus their thinking on the tasks they are undertaking, empowering them to reflect on what they have learnt, enabling them to identify their learning needs, encouraging them to improve their self-directed learning and providing them with the opportunity to critically evaluate their work.

WHAT ARE THE USES OF PORTFOLIOS?

Portfolios create links between assessment and learning. This is particularly useful when students are required to reflect on their learning, provide examples of situations in which they applied knowledge learnt, uncover the kinds of questions that lead to changing their attitude, make explicit connections between their learning priorities and the objectives of their course and use feedback to improve their performance. In this way, portfolios can be used as evidence of progress and the ability to achieve specific outcomes. A portfolio may comprise a number of learning activities (see Box 9.1). *Note that most of the discussion in the chapter centres on the component of the portfolio that is most useful in the early years of your course: the reflective journal.*

BOX 9.1 Learning activities that may be included in a portfolio:

Case studies/case reports
— learning experiences acquired from clinical cases
— questions raised in the learning process
— approaches used to foster deep learning
— commentaries on journal articles, clinical cases, evidence-based papers or review articles
— critical evaluation of published works
— evidence-based practices used to address particular situations
— videotapes of consultations
— reflections on difficulties and successes during clinical rotations
— online resources identified and used in learning
— time management strategies and methods used to implement these strategies
— examples of learning issues showing construction of new information, use of flow charts, mechanisms and concept maps.

PORTFOLIOS IN A PBL COURSE

Portfolios have a number of uses in a PBL course.

1 ASSESSMENT IN THE CLINICAL YEARS

Portfolios can be used in the clinical years to establish links between students' learning and assessment. The feedback and comments provided by the mentor are important in improving students' learning and helping them deal with their weaknesses.

Portfolios can also be used to assess areas that are difficult to assess, for example:

1 attitudes
2 personal attributes
3 teamwork
4 reflective learning.

Portfolios can include:

- case reports
- critical analyses of clinical cases
- descriptions of learning experiences
- videotapes of clinical consultations
- construction of management plans
- follow-up reports of patients seen before and after a clinical procedure/surgery
- reflection on concepts learnt and how to use knowledge learnt in similar situations
- interpretation of patients' laboratory results and other investigations in the light of patients' problems, history and clinical examinations
- literature reviews and evidence-based practices.

2 DEVELOPING SELF-DIRECTED LEARNING SKILLS

Students can use portfolios to:

- define research questions
- demonstrate how to search for information and use resources effectively
- develop the skill of construction of new information
- learn how to identify learning needs, plan learning and evaluate progress.

3 SELF-EMPOWERMENT AND DEVELOPING REFLECTIVE LEARNING SKILLS

By using a portfolio students become:

- goal-centred
- strategic learners
- focused on acquiring new skills
- skilful in reflecting on concepts learnt and in applying new information
- able to overcome challenges in clinical learning.

REFLECTIVE JOURNALS IN A PBL COURSE

A reflective journal can help the learner to:

- define overall goals and identify objectives
- specify areas of strength and skills they need to develop
- construct an action plan to achieve their goals
- reflect upon learning experiences and the challenges they face

- include examples of situations that helped them foster their learning
- demonstrate that they have handled a wide range of tasks to deepen their learning
- show the range of resources and strategies used to gather information
- document their experiences and areas of growth
- identify types of support they need to develop their skills/competencies
- include observations, clinical scenarios, or clinical challenges and the learning issues that arise from these situations
- ask questions that can reinforce their objectives
- focus their approach and readjust their actions
- set their learning objectives for the coming period
- think about future areas of development
- reflect upon observations in clinical classes
- evaluate progress and achievements
- enable their tutor to get to know more about them.

HOW DO I CONSTRUCT MY REFLECTIVE JOURNAL?

Constructing a reflective journal requires a lot of thought. Your faculty will provide you with clear instructions and a number of probing questions to stimulate your thinking. Use these questions plus those I list below to scaffold the construction of your journal. See also the example pages of a reflective journal on p. 160–2.

Goals and objectives
- What are my goals for this semester?
- What am I trying to achieve?
- What is my plan to achieve these goals?
- What are my areas of strength and what skills do I need to develop?
- What should I do to develop these skills?
- Do I need help? What type of help do I need? What type of support is available to me?

Time management
- Why do I need to plan my time?
- What approach should I use to organise my time?
- What are my priorities?
- What are the sources of time wasting?
- What strategies do I use to minimise my time wasting?

Learning resources
- What type of resources am I using?
- Do I use my resources effectively? How?
- What changes do I need to make to improve my learning from these resources?
- Am I clear about my search questions before using my resources?
- Do I use tables, flow charts, diagrams, mechanisms, simple models or analogies to construct new information?

Problem-based learning tutorials
- How is PBL different from what I used to do?
- What is my role in PBL tutorials?
- Do I understand what I need to do to achieve my goals?
- Am I a regular contributor to the discussion in my group? What is preventing me from contributing more?
- What roles did I take on this week?

- What roles did I avoid taking on? Why?
- How can I improve my skills in these areas?
- Do I need help in any area?
- How can my contribution to my PBL group become more useful to the group dynamics?
- What will make our group work more efficiently and effectively?
- How do I feel about this experience?
- What can I change to better support myself and other members in the group?

Skills and learning style
- What type of skills do I need in a PBL course?
- What type of skills do I have?
- What type of skills do I need to develop?
- Do I need to change my learning style?
- What exactly do I need to change?
- How does this connect with previous experiences?
- How do these changes help me improve my learning?
- How can I acquire these new skills? What is my plan?

Organisation and computer skills
- Have I organised my computer files?
- What approach should I use in this process?
- Is it easy to find a folder or a summary note?
- What changes should I consider to improve my organisational skills?
- How has this situation enhanced my learning?

Lectures and practical classes
- What should I do to get the best out of lectures, clinical rounds, small-group discussion and clinical seminars?
- How can I use the information learnt from these settings to add to my learning?
- Do I integrate the information learnt from clinical settings with knowledge learnt from basic sciences? How?
- What questions do these clinical cases raise?
- How can I use knowledge/skills learnt from practical classes to add to my learning?

Clinical sessions and evidence-based medicine
- How can the skills I have learnt in the clinical classes be integrated with knowledge learnt from basic sciences?
- Do I use the clinical classes/rounds/seminars effectively to enhance my learning?
- What changes should I make to enhance my learning from these classes?
- Do I use evidence-based strategies as I learn a new topic?
- How can I improve my evidence-based practices?
- How can I integrate evidence-based practices in my learning?

Evaluation
- Do I evaluate my work regularly?
- What resources can I use in my evaluation?
- What parameters do I use in my evaluation?
- How can I improve my evaluation process?
- How can I use my evaluation to further my learning and achievements?
- Have I achieved my goals?

WHAT ARE THE ADVANTAGES OF REFLECTIVE JOURNALS?

Current studies show that reflective journals can improve:
- personal and professional growth
- engagement in the PBL process and collaborative learning
- ability to acquire new learning skills
- learning from experiences
- thinking, reflective and analytical skills
- working towards particular goals.

WHAT ARE THE LIMITATIONS?

1 Students may believe that recording their reflections is not helpful and a waste of time because: (1) they have not used reflective journals during their high school education or in other university courses, (2) they were not adequately informed about or trained to create reflective journals, (3) they believe that their learning should focus on factual knowledge rather than reflective experiences, (4) they do not like self-evaluation or thinking about deficiencies and skills they need to develop, and (5) they do not know how to analyse their learning or assess their learning experiences. However, there is evidence that training students in workshops to construct their reflective journals, use probing questions and analyse their learning experiences can help them use reflective journals effectively.

2 There has been little work published on the validity and educational uses of reflective journals. However, it is clear from student feedback that reflective journals assist them in areas such as:
— time management
— contribution to PBL tutorials
— acquiring new skills and prioritising
— development of planning skills.

3 Students may raise concerns about the degree of detail they need to include and whether there are ethical or confidentiality implications.

4 The success of reflection depends on the reflective skills of learners. But there is evidence that reflective skills can be dramatically improved through training, practice writing, feedback and tutor support.

WHAT STUDENTS SAY ABOUT THEIR REFLECTIVE JOURNALS

These are quotes compiled from first-year medical students.

'… In the beginning I was not sure what I should write and how to construct my reflective journal. The guidelines provided by my tutor and the key questions given helped me a lot in designing my journal.'

'If you do not start constructing your reflective journal early in the semester, it will become very difficult to start this process and you will delay it week after week. Once you start your journal, you will enjoy doing it.'

'… the learning I gained from my reflective journal is beyond description. It turned my attitude about the PBL course into an enjoyable experience. These journals in fact helped me to disclose myself, and explore areas of strengths and skills I need to develop. Such reflections gave me the power to examine deep inside me, think about my attitude, work on developing new habits and become aware of my priorities and the skills I need to develop.'

'The comments and feedback I received from my tutor on my journal helped me a lot to negotiate areas I need help in and the kind of support I need to improve my learning.'

HOW TO GET THE BEST OUT OF YOUR REFLECTIVE JOURNAL

These twelve tips will help you construct your reflective journal.

TIP 1 DO IT NOW

Get started. Do it now. Make your reflective journal one of your learning priorities. There is no doubt that you get more by doing it now. Focusing on your reflective journal and working on it regularly is not easy, but the consequences of not doing so can be much worse than the challenge of starting.

By starting work on your reflective journals you will feel better about yourself and more confident in progressing with it. The thoughts and ideas that will come to you, and keep you engaged as you go through the probing questions, will energise you.

TIP 2 PROGRAM YOUR MIND FOR SUCCESS

The aim of the reflective journal is to stimulate your experiential learning, promote deep learning and encourage your reflection. Reflection can stimulate the development of learning that impacts on your behaviour, performance and skills. Therefore, you need to reflect and construct your journal in a powerful way that targets success. Do not treat it as a routine job.

When you program your mind for success you will:
• Enjoy doing your journal.
• Target deep learning.
• Focus on your goals and objectives.
• Recognise areas of weakness and gaps in your learning that need further work.

TIP 3 KNOW WHAT IS NEEDED FROM YOU

Some courses provide training for students and also for supervisors, mentors and tutors. The aims are to: (1) ensure that students know how to develop their reflective journals and understand exactly what is needed from them, (2) provide students with support from adequately trained staff, and (3) provide information to tutors about the uses of journals in training, assessment and providing constructive feedback.

If the training program in your faculty is not adequate, read the guidelines provided and focus on the:
• purpose of your journal
• style recommended
• probing and facilitating questions
• focus and the scope of the journal
• evaluation criteria
• time available for you to construct your journal.

TIP 4 BE CLEAR ABOUT YOUR GOALS AND PURPOSE

When you are clear about your goals and purpose you will:
- focus your reflections on specific outcomes
- use your reflective journal effectively to deepen your learning
- target problem–based experiential learning
- demonstrate the value of providing evidence to strengthen your reflections
- sharpen your focus.

TIP 5 BE CREATIVE

One of the aims of the reflective journal is to facilitate links between theory and practice, demonstrating evidence of deep learning, appropriate selection of material and showing how the experience helped your personal and professional development. Reflective skills are essential to construct educationally useful journals. With creative reflection you:
- show your active role in transition from high school; your adaptation to a new environment
- demonstrate critical analysis of your experience (for example, the use of knowledge in the PBL context)
- assess the educational usefulness of tasks you undertake
- discover gaps in your experience and point to resources to use to enrich your experience
- develop the reasoning and thinking processes to identify your learning needs
- show insight into the challenges you face.

TIP 6 DO NOT EXAGGERATE

The primary objective of a reflective journal is to help you achieve personal and professional development so you need to be realistic and aware of the value of evidence in strengthening your reflections. In fact accurate reflections:
- match with what you want to achieve over a specific period of time
- help you plan to reach your target
- guide you to go deeper into yourself to explore your fears, challenges and dreams.

    Through this exploration you will be able to:
- develop your reflective insights and analytical skills
- match the learning needs and competencies you have developed at a particular stage.

TIP 7 PROVIDE EXAMPLES

By providing examples in your journal, you will strengthen the evidence for your argument. Examples could include:
- critical incidents in PBL tutorials where you felt group discussion lacked elaboration, interaction, participation or motivation and how such incidents inhibited the learning process or affected the group function
- the discussion of a PBL case (problem) was not to the depth you needed to achieve and your group members left the tutorial unsure about their learning issues. You felt it was a challenging experience and were not sure how to search for your learning

- two students in your group come to PBL tutorials with a lot of notes. They read from their notes or copies of textbooks instead of reporting information or sharing ideas with other members. You wonder whether this is the right approach for learning.

But providing examples is not the primary purpose of the journal. What is more important is how you see the incident, what type of questions you raise, what your perception is, how you work on the problem, what your approach is, how you progress, whether you consult with other people, how the experience is useful to you and in what way. Discussing such questions in relation to your example will add useful information to what you are constructing in your journal.

Providing examples in your reflective journal will:
- enable you to dig deeper into different aspects of the challenges you are facing
- allow you to reflect upon possible contributing factors, circumstances, options available, responsibilities, information needed, impact on you and others, and learning experiences
- make you more aware of the differences between traditional teaching and student-centred/self-directed learning and the changes you need to make to your learning style to suit PBL.

TIP 8 FOCUS ON YOUR LEARNING EXPERIENCES

Without reflection, the learning process will become limited and static. By writing about your learning experiences and recording your reflections, you add new dimensions to your learning. However, a journal is more than a simple description of incidents. The aim is to go beyond description and critically reflect on your learning experiences:
- Explore your personal beliefs about the situation.
- Critically analyse the situation.
- Reflect on your own actions, decisions and the knowledge learnt from the situation.
- Examine your willingness to change your beliefs or actions.
- Examine the value of these experiences.

TIP 9 SHOW HOW YOUR GOALS ARE ACHIEVED

Defining your learning goals and what you need to achieve is an essential step. Your reflective journal can tell the story of your success and the different stages you went through to achieve your goals. Achieving a particular goal is not the end of the story: it is a continuous process. Reaching a particular goal raises new challenges and keeps you engaged. In your reflective journal you can:
- critically discuss the procedures and processes you have considered to achieve your goals
- evaluate your approaches and other options you have
- discuss challenges you faced during the journey.

TIP 10 EVALUATE YOUR PROGRESS

Your reflective journal can be an excellent tool for assessing your progress as well as your personal and professional growth. This will be useful to you as well as to the faculty. There are a number of parameters you may use to evaluate your progress:

- commitment to your work
- development of your critical and analytical skills
- ability to reduce the gap between theory and practice
- thought processes and quality of questions you raise in discussion
- quality of evidence you provide to support your arguments
- ability to achieve your goals within the timeframe of your plan
- ability to acquire new skills and develop competencies
- changes in attitude and behaviour.

Your reflective journal may not cover all these areas. However, it can be a useful tool in self-evaluation, and help you focus on your goals and monitor your progress.

TIP 11 TURN IT INTO AN ENJOYABLE EXPERIENCE

Unless your reflective journal is perceived by you to be relevant and useful to your learning, it will be of limited value and working on it will be a waste of time. There is no doubt that the time you spend on constructing your journal cannot be underestimated. However, there is evidence that when you are clear about the process and understand the purpose, content and structure you will be able to manage your time and enjoy the whole experience.

Turning it into an enjoyable experience will depend on your:
- perceptions of learning and the usefulness of reflection
- willingness to assess your skills and develop new skills.
- realisation of the personal and professional learning needs necessary for your course
- awareness of the learning skills needed in a PBL curriculum
- willingness to enjoy your learning and turn it into a life-long experience
- willingness to use your reflection in a constructive manner that will have a major impact on you in the long term.

TIP 12 ASK FOR FEEDBACK

It will be impossible for you to improve your work without clear feedback from your tutor. Always ask for their recommendations to help you be more efficient. By showing your willingness to improve and your interest in knowing the views of people around you, you are really seeking excellence in your performance, demonstrating interest in learning new skills and confirming that you possess the attitude and commitment of a good learner. Use the feedback provided by your tutor to:
- focus your purpose
- identify your priorities
- enhance your personal and professional skills
- improve the quality of your critical reflections and your actions
- maximise your learning potential
- analyse situations and use critical incidents to foster deep learning.

CONCLUSIONS

The process of reflective learning and constructing portfolios and reflective journals is time consuming but rewarding. Reflective journals allow learners to review their experiences, and personal and professional growth. They are a useful tool to enhance critical thinking and allow learners to evaluate their behaviour and practices. The twelve tips and the examples provided in this chapter will help you develop your own reflective journals and portfolios. I strongly believe that practice is the best of all instructors and is the only way to make quality improvements. Start your reflective journal today.

EVIDENCE-BASED LEARNING
Portfolio as a method for continuous assessment in an undergraduate health education programme

A portfolio assessment system has been introduced into a biomedical science programme to promote both continuous learning and deep approaches to learning. Attention has been focused on creating harmony between the assessment system and the PBL curriculum of the programme. Biomedicine and laboratory work are central in the curriculum. The portfolio included evidence of laboratory work, personal reflections and certificates from the PBL tutor. The portfolio was assessed on three occasions over 20 weeks. The grades were 'pass' or 'fail'. The tutor certificate appeared to be a crucial part of the portfolio since a 'fail' in this part usually led to an overall 'fail'. Both students and teachers were concerned about ensuring that enough factual knowledge, as measured by a traditional test, had been achieved. The agreement was good enough for the pass or fail level but some expected differences were found at the detailed level. The course, including the portfolio, was evaluated orally during weekly whole-group meetings and using a questionnaire at the end. The students felt comfortable with the portfolio system and preferred it to a traditional test. The teachers felt that they needed to develop their teacher-student discussion skills and to improve their feedback on the reflections. Peer assessment between students is proposed as a line of action to enhance the credibility of the crucial tutor certificate. The portfolio might be an efficient tool for the students to concentrate their efforts on the most central concepts of medical laboratory work. The model will be developed through further discussions and better consensus among faculty.

Thome G, Hovenberg H, Edgren G. Med Teach 2006; 28(6):e171–e176. Adapted with permission from the publisher.
For more information: http://www.tandf.co.uk/journals/titles/0142159X.asp

FURTHER READING
BOOKS
Klenowski V. Developing portfolios for learning and assessment: processes and principles. London: RoutledgeFalmer; 2002.

ARTICLES AND RESEARCH PAPERS
Amsellem-Ouazana D, Van Pee D, Godin V. Use of portfolios as a learning and assessment tool in a surgical practical session of urology during undergraduate medical training. Med Teach 2006; 28(4):356–359.
Driessen EW, Overeem K, van Tartwijk J, et al. Validity of portfolio assessment: which qualities determine ratings? Med Educ 2006; 40(9):862–866.
Driessen EW, van Tartwijk J, Overeem K, et al. Conditions for successful reflective use of portfolios in undergraduate medical education. Med Educ 2005; 39(12):1230–1235.

Garrett BM, Jackson C. A mobile clinical e-portfolio for nursing and medical students, using wireless personal digital assistants (PDAs). Nurse Educ Today 2006; 26(8):647–654.

McMullan M, Endacott R, Gray MA, et al. Portfolios and assessment of competence: a review of the literature. J Adv Nurs 2003; 41(3):283–294.

Scholes J, Webb C, Gray M, et al. Making portfolios work in practice. J Adv Nurs 2004; 46(6):595–603.

Thome G, Hovenberg H, Edgren G. Portfolio as a method for continuous assessment in an undergraduate health education programme. Med Teach 2006; 28(6):e171–e176.

EXAMPLE OF A REFLECTIVE JOURNAL

I have enclosed a reflective journal, 15 days in length. You can make changes to this blueprint to create your own structure. Construct a new page for every day of your semester.

Day 1
It starts with a goal
Main focus: I have a goal
Questions to think about: What are my goals? What is the big picture? What are the goals I would like to achieve by the end of this semester?

What skills and qualities would I like to achieve? What is the big picture?

I have a goal and I would like to be clear about the purpose of my study and what exactly I want to achieve by the end of this semester.

For the other days I've suggested a focus for each and questions to think about:

Day 2
What is this semester about?
Main focus: I need to know
Questions to think about: What are the objectives of this semester? What is PBL all about? How is PBL different from what I used to do?

Day 3
Understanding my roles
Main focus: PBL is student-centred learning
Questions to think about: What are my roles in PBL tutorials? What roles and skills do I need to develop?

Day 4
What matters most
Main focus: Knowing my priorities
Questions to think about: What are my learning priorities? Do my priorities match with the course objectives and my learning needs?

Day 5
Think planning
Main focus: Planning is vital
Questions to think about: What is my plan? How can I place my priorities into a workable plan? What is my timeframe?

Day 6
Experiencing small-group learning
Main focus: Enjoying what I am doing
Questions to think about: What do I enjoy in PBL tutorials? What are the things I do not enjoy? Why?

Day 7
Cultivating my skills
Main focus: Investing in my skills
Questions to think about: What are the skills I need to develop? How can I develop these skills? What resources are available to me?

Day 8
Growing through challenges
Main focus: Turning challenges into success
Questions to think about: What are the challenges I face at this stage? How are these challenges affecting my plans?

Day 9
What makes my group function well?
Main focus: Success of my group adds to my success
Questions to think about: How do I feel about my PBL group? What am I doing to enhance group dynamics?

Day 10
My self-directed learning
Main focus: Mastering self-directed learning is one of my priorities
Questions to think about: Do I know how to search my learning issues? How do I choose my resources? What strategies do I use in my search?

Day 11
Peer feedback
Main focus: There are benefits from sharing views with others
Questions to think about: How do others in my group see PBL tutorials? How do they prepare their learning issues and search for new information? Is there anything to share or learn from this discussion?

Day 12
Self-assessment
Main focus: There are no shortcuts to excellence
Questions to think about: What is my assessment of my work and contribution to PBL tutorials? What areas do I need to improve? How?

Day 13
Dealing with setback
Main focus: Turning obstacles into opportunities for success
Questions to think about: How can I deal with my setback? How can I approach this challenge? What are my fears? What are the sources of my strength?

Day 14
Receiving feedback from my tutor
Main focus: I need feedback

Questions to think about: How does my tutor see my contribution to the PBL tutorials? How can I use their recommendations to improve my skills?

Day 15
Constructing mechanisms
Main focus: Knowing the pathogenesis allows better understanding
Questions to think about: What do I know about mechanisms? How can I share in developing them with others in PBL tutorials? How can we improve our mechanism? What do we need to change?

PART THREE

ASSESSMENT

CHAPTER 10

Assessment in a problem-based learning curriculum

> Assessment of cognitive skills of students is not only the most difficult but also the most neglected area in the assessment of medical competence. **JOHN MARSHALL**

INTRODUCTION

The educational principles on which most problem–based learning (PBL) courses are based are: the use of problems to acquire a knowledge base that is easier to retain than simple factual information; self-directed learning and communication skills; integration of basic and clinical sciences; small-group learning and collaboration and an emphasis on community-related issues in the curriculum. Because PBL assessment needs to match the philosophy of the curriculum and reflect its educational outcomes it requires more complex outcomes than simply the ability of examinees to recall information. But although acquiring new medical knowledge and improving personal skills are expected outcomes these should not be the main focus of assessment. Ideally, assessment targets the ability of students to develop new professional habits (what they do habitually even when not observed), to use and apply knowledge learnt to real-life situations, to solve problems and deal with uncertainty as well as to become responsible for their self-directed learning. Using appropriate assessment tools to test each of these competencies/skills is essential. In fact, one of the reasons for using a wide range of assessment tools such as written tests, clinical simulations, peer assessment, self-assessment, tutor assessment and a portfolio is to ensure that different competencies have been adequately addressed. Using a range of tools can compensate for limitations and flaws in any one method.

AIMS OF ASSESSMENT

Assessment plays an integral role in helping students identify and respond to their learning needs. Other aims of assessment in a PBL curriculum are to:
- optimise the capability of learners by providing motivation and direction for further learning
- ensure that students have acquired the knowledge, skills and competencies highlighted in the curriculum for each stage in their course
- identify incompetent students and ensure that all graduates are competent and able to manage patients' problems without causing harm and are able to demonstrate professional behaviour
- judge the adequacy of the clinical program and the structure of the curriculum.

SUMMATIVE ASSESSMENT

The two main terms in relation to assessment that you will become aware of during your course are summative and formative assessments (Table 10.1). *Summative assessment* covers the skills, knowledge and attitudes that you have acquired during the semester or year. The aims of summative assessment are to:
- ensure that you have achieved these competencies/skills
- determine your effectiveness and level of achievement
- officially declare that you have fulfilled the requirements of a particular stage in your learning and that you can progress to the next stage
- provide the entrance requirements to a higher educational institution.
  An ideal summative assessment should:
- match the students' expectations and what they have learnt during the course/semester
- cover competencies, skills and knowledge highlighted in the curriculum
- use a wide range of assessment tools, for example, multiple-choice questions (MCQs), extended-matching questions (EMQs), PBL-style questions, short-answer questions (SAQs), portfolios, tutor reports, objective structured clinical examination (OSCE)
- match the style of the formative assessment (see below)
- focus on understanding and application of knowledge, skills and competencies rather than regurgitation of factual knowledge
- comprise questions that are valid and reliable.

TABLE 10.1 Main differences between summative and formative assessments

	Summative assessment	Formative assessment
Purpose	Provision of an overall judgement of students' performance so they can proceed to the next stage, graduate, be licensed to practise or be deemed not fit to practise and be expelled from the course	Guides future learning Provides reassurance Promotes students' reflection
Outcomes	Officially declare that students have fulfilled the requirements of a particular stage and can progress to the next	Orients the learner and helps to focus their learning strategies. Reinforces students' intrinsic motivation
Feedback	Summative assessment is usually not followed by a feedback session	Feedback is provided after formative assessment to improve students' learning

FORMATIVE ASSESSMENT

The main objectives of *formative assessment* are to guide future learning, provide reassurance, promote students' reflection, and foster students' learning about concepts raised in the curriculum. Formative assessment does not count as a hurdle and its results are not added to the summative total final score. Other objectives of formative assessment are to:
- allow students to review what they have learnt, test their understanding and receive feedback from the tutors to improve their performance—this is possible because it is built into the coursework

- provide students with the opportunity to understand the assessment requirements, competencies and skills to be tested in the summative assessment
- provide students with the opportunity to monitor their progress and to focus on competencies, knowledge and skills they need to acquire
- encourage students to establish links between learning and assessment and change their learning style to suit the needs of the course and become strategic learners.

Formative assessment can take different forms, including:
- self- and peer assessment in PBL tutorials
- self-assessment by using an online bank of questions
- assignments
- quizzes undertaken during the semester
- self-assessment by using interactive multimedia
- mid-semester examination.

In many schools formative assessment takes the form of quizzes or mid-semester examinations. Immediately after completing one of these assessments, students meet with representatives from the examination team to discuss their answers. Such meetings allow students to reflect on their answers, discuss what they understood, identify gaps in their knowledge and highlight areas they misunderstood as well as learn through discussion with other students. This approach helps students acquire new knowledge, deepen their understanding and learn to apply knowledge to address examination questions.

Feedback sessions in formative assessment
Feedback sessions:
- inform students about their strengths and weaknesses
- allow students to foster their skills and focus on their goals
- motivate students to explore the issues assessed and deepen their understanding.

COMPETENCIES IN MEDICINE

> Competence in medicine is the habitual and judicious use of communication, knowledge, technical skills, clinical reasoning, emotions, values, and reflection in daily practice for the benefit of individuals and communities being served. DAVID C LEACH

According to the Accreditation Council for Graduate Medical Education (ACGME), there are six areas of competency to be measured in resident training: (1) patient care (including clinical reasoning), (2) medical knowledge, (3) practice-based learning and improvement (including information management), (4) interpersonal and communication skills, (5) professionalism, and (6) system-based practice (including health economics and teamwork). For more information see the ACGME document (http://www.acgme.org/acWebsite/irc_competencies.pdf).

Competencies identified for undergraduate medical courses may vary from those identified for resident training. However, they share the same concepts and are adjusted to the stage of the curriculum. Each competence highlights a number of skills that can be measured by using appropriate tools: for example, medical knowledge may be tested by using multiple-choice questions (MCQs), oral examinations and short-answer questions (SAQs) while clinical reasoning may be tested by using objective structured clinical examination (OSCE) and PBL-style questions. This approach to assessment matches the changes introduced in the curriculum and the philosophy of PBL. See Chs 11 and 12 for more details.

ASSESSMENT TOOLS

The usefulness of a particular assessment tool is determined by a number of factors including: (1) reliability (the degree to which the measurement is accurate and reproducible), (2) validity (whether the assessment measures what it claims to measure), (3) impact on future learning and personal development, (4) face validity (the degree to which questions match with students' expectation), and (5) the capability of the tool to examine more than one competence/skill. The tools used in assessment in a PBL curriculum can be summarised as:

1 MULTIPLE-CHOICE QUESTIONS (MCQs)

Multiple-choice questions have been extensively used in the assessment of students in medical and other healthcare courses. MCQs are widely used in examinations for a number of reasons:
- They enable educators to test a broad range of topics in the curriculum.
- Marking of MCQs is cost-effective as they are usually marked electronically.
- The results can be statistically analysed to provide information on facility index (degree of difficulty of questions) and the discrimination power of test items.
- They are suitable for examinations intended for thousands of examinees.

However, the educational goals of traditional MCQs are to test factual knowledge rather than test deeper understanding or the use of information learnt in real-life situations. Traditional MCQs do not test cognitive skills; many of them test 'the small print' in textbooks. Other limitations of traditional MCQs are: (1) the use of these questions can interfere with students' learning process and force them to focus on details in lectures and textbooks rather than the desired skills embedded in PBL, (2) traditional MCQs do not match with the philosophy of integration of knowledge, critical thinking and weighing evidence for each hypothesis, and (3) traditional MCQs have limited validity for measuring the application of knowledge.

The new generations of MCQs such as scenario-based multiple-choice questions (see Appendix D for examples) can test a wide range of skills such as: (1) analytical skills, (2) problem-solving skills, (3) integration of knowledge, (4) justification and clinical reasoning, and (5) application of knowledge. The use of a scenario as the stem of the question enables the construction of questions that are free from grammatical clues (such as 'may', 'may be', 'never', 'always', 'usually', 'all'), imprecise terms and trivialities or small print in textbooks. Usually the scenario is followed by five items; students have to choose only one item for their answer. This type of MCQ is often called 'single-best answer'.

2 EXTENDED-MATCHING QUESTIONS (EMQs)

Extended-matching questions are MCQs organised into sets that use one list of options for all items in the set. EMQs test application of knowledge and deeper understanding by using 4 to 5 case scenarios addressing one theme. For example, EMQs could test knowledge about the different mechanisms by which antihypertensive drugs work, the drug interaction, or decision making regarding the drug of choice in a number of case scenarios where a number of factors could affect the management options (see Appendix D).

3 SHORT-ANSWER QUESTIONS (SAQs)

These questions test factual knowledge. They have a number of limitations: (1) do not allow testing of cognitive skills, (2) allow testing of only a few topics per unit of time (possibly 6 questions and each question is answered in 10 minutes), and (3) marking can be time consuming. Although SAQs may be used in the early years of the medical course, they are not favoured in the clinical years (see Appendix D).

4 PBL-STYLE QUESTIONS

These questions suit the PBL structure. The questions might test a number of educational objectives including: applying knowledge to real situations, generating hypotheses, weighing evidence for and against each hypothesis, constructing mechanisms that demonstrate pathogenesis and integration of knowledge. The blueprint for this tool is that questions start with a case scenario followed by a question addressing one of the educational objectives. The limitations of this assessment are: (1) does not allow testing of fine detail, (2) creating these questions is demanding, and (3) marking the answers is time consuming (see Appendix D).

5 MODIFIED-ESSAY QUESTIONS (MEQs)

This type of question has been widely used in medical and other healthcare schools. An MEQ consists of a brief case scenario followed by two or three questions. The questions are designed to assess application of knowledge, interpretation of findings, generation of hypotheses or provision of a justification.

6 CONSTRUCTED-RESPONSE QUESTIONS (CRQs)

These are open-ended, short-answer questions that can be used in summative and formative assessment. Questions measure application of knowledge, testing cognitive skills as well as understanding content knowledge. CRQs use a range of stimuli to facilitate this educational objective. For example, the stem of the question may be followed by a timeline, table, graph, chart, diagram, radiology film, pathology specimen, or an image of anatomical structures. Model answers are usually prepared by the questions' authors. Marking these questions is graded against specific criteria. The marking system allows for partial credit (see Appendix D).

7 TAG TESTS

This type of assessment is used in practical examinations. It involves the tagging of dissected cadavers, body organs, pathology specimens or radiological films and asking questions related to the tagged structure. Students may answer by writing two or three sentences. Some schools use MCQs in combination with a tagged structure.

8 TUTOR ASSESSMENT

This assessment is discussed in detail on pp. 172–3.

9 CLINICAL SIMULATIONS

The hallmark of clinical simulations is authentic simulations that are reflective of real-world practices. For example, clinical simulations can be used to assist students in breaking bad news to patients. This might be done by constructing a case scenario and training a simulated patient (a surrogate patient) to portray a woman at risk of hereditary breast cancer. Students are given a task such as, 'Break the bad news to a 45-year-old patient who has been confirmed to be at high risk of developing breast cancer'.

This examination would focus on issues such as:

* interpersonal skills (e.g. empathy)
* communication skills (e.g. appropriate use of verbal and non-verbal cues)
* ability to respond appropriately to patient's questions
* ability to provide information to the patient (e.g. support available to the patient, possible options for the management plan)
* ability to construct student-drawn pedigrees for the patient.

The use of simulation in formative and summative assessment has a number of advantages:
* Teaching and training is done in a non-threatening environment.
* Procedures are taught in a safe environment with no risk to patient or student.
* Procedures are repeated as necessary to achieve optimal performance.
* Students can receive feedback from their tutor, peers, and the surrogate patient.
* The process can be adjusted to suit the appropriate stage of the curriculum.
* The process compensates for declining numbers of accessible inpatients.

However, simulation centres and clinical skills laboratories are expensive to build and equip and require substantial funding. The clinical skills laboratories may comprise: (1) simulation products such as an injection trainer, knot-tying trainer, skin pad-wound closure, suture practice leg, suture practice arm, injection model, abdominal palpation model, gynaecological simulator, pelvic examination simulator, catheterisation simulator, adult airway management, spinal injection simulator, and whole body manikin; (2) CD-ROMs and interactive programs; and (3) surrogate patients. Patient simulation can be used in OSCE stations (see below), highlighting specific educational tasks.

10 OBJECTIVE STRUCTURED CLINICAL EXAMINATION (OSCE)

This examination comprises a series of timed stations at which students are asked to complete a task. In some stations, students may be observed by one or two examiners while carrying out the task. The OSCE is structured so that questions have a defined marking system with predetermined answers and pass/fail criteria. The OSCE assesses specific clinical skills such as: (1) taking a medical history, (2) providing a differential diagnosis, (3) interpreting investigation results, (4) constructing a management plan, and (5) examining a patient.

11 STUDENT'S LOGBOOK

The use of logbooks can provide insight into the practical activities undertaken by students during their clinical rotations. However, there are a number of limitations for logbooks:
* there is often an inherent bias in self-reporting
* some students may not be sufficiently motivated to complete their logbooks
* students may fabricate entries to achieve a higher grade. However, most schools using logbooks have systems to detect such behaviour.

12 ORAL EXAMINATION

Oral examinations can provide students with the opportunity to elaborate on their knowledge. They also allow examiners to dig deeper and ensure that students understand the concept discussed. One of the limitations of oral examinations is that students have to deal with different styles of questioning: some examiners may be supportive facilitators; others may use an aggressive or confrontational style.

13 THE TRIPLE-JUMP EXAMINATION (TJ)

The triple-jump examination assesses: (1) students' clinical problem-solving processes, and (2) students' competence in self-directed learning. The test comprises three steps:

Step 1: Student reads written problem and discusses the problem with the tutor. Student then selects some tasks related to the case for further learning and decides on key issues to be researched.

Step 2: Student uses relevant resources and collects the information needed. They construct the new information to address the issues they have identified.

Step 3: Student reports back to the tutor, presents their findings and provides a summary for the problem. The tutor provides feedback on the way in which the student addressed the problem.

The PBL tutor might also use the triple-jump examination to assess three or four students by asking them to work together on a problem and report back to the group.

14 THE MULTIPLE MINI-INTERVIEW (MMI)

Multiple mini-interviews are a recent development and have been used in student selection to medical schools. They have also been used to predict students' performance in the early years of their course. The MMI can be used in the assessment of students' non-cognitive skills such as interpersonal skills, cultural sensitivity, teamwork, empathy, communication skills and professionalism. For this assessment, candidates are guided through 10 interviews, each 10 minutes long. At each interview, the candidate is presented with a brief case scenario designed to assess one of the non-cognitive skills. There is no specific correct answer; the candidate is expected to discuss the case scenario and what they would do if they faced such a situation. More research is needed to assess the validity and reliability of the multiple mini-interview.

15 THE MINI-CLINICAL EVALUATION EXERCISE (MINI-CEX)

The mini-clinical evaluation exercise was initially developed by the American Board of Internal Medicine (ABIM) to assess residents' clinical performance. It is currently used by several universities in the US, Canada and Europe to assess the clinical performance of medical students.

The test is a focused, brief and observed clinical encounter followed by immediate feedback provided by the examiner. The encounter can occur in various settings— outpatient, inpatient, emergency department. Students are expected to complete 3 or 4 mini-CEXs. Each encounter is with one patient and students are expected to complete each encounter in 15–20 minutes. An examiner is present for each encounter and assesses students using a standard mini-CEX form covering a number of domains—medical interviewing, clinical examination, humanistic component, professionalism, clinical judgement, organisation skills, counselling skills, efficacy and overall clinical performance.

16 PEER ASSESSMENT

Peer assessment has been used in higher education for a number of years and has been shown to enhance the development of self-motivation, responsibility and reflective learning. In PBL it is used as one of the formative assessment tools. It involves examining a peer's work and comparing it against a predefined criteria agreed by the group members and the faculty. Schools using this type of assessment report that students enjoy the process of peer assessment and find it fair and useful to their learning. PBL group members may need to identify the ground rules before implementing peer assessment so that the process is constructive.

17 PORTFOLIOS

This assessment tool is discussed in full in Ch 9.

ASSESSMENT BY TUTOR

Assessment in PBL tutorials can include a combination of methods involving elements of peer, self- and tutor assessment. The peer and self-assessment elements are usually part of the formative assessment, while the tutor's assessment is only summative. However, some schools have successfully used tutor's assessment as both a formative and summative tool. Tutor assessment consists of a standardised report, completed by the tutor, and tutor's feedback for each student. Such assessment is particularly useful because it enables the assessment of areas that cannot be examined by conventional methods. For example:
- listening skills and interaction with other members of the group
- personal attributes
- dealing with uncertainties and handling challenging situations
- sharing knowledge with other members
- contributing to group dynamics and group success
- demonstrating professional values, for example, reliability and respect for other group members
- demonstrating the skills encouraged in small groups and PBL curricula.

The standardised report used for this purpose must be well designed. Schools using this method often follow these principles:
- The report is based on specific criteria related to the objectives of the course.
- Early in the course, students are informed about the report structure and the criteria to be addressed, for example, communication and interpersonal skills, problem-solving skills and self-directed learning.
- The report is easy to use and implement. New tutors are usually trained to use the report and to provide constructive feedback to their students.
- The report assesses students' performance over a period of time, for example, 5–6 weeks (sustained performance rather than snapshot obtained during an examination).

Other uses of this assessment are:
- identifying underperforming students and providing them with appropriate support

- highlighting skills and attitudes encouraged in the course
- giving feedback to help students progress, work on their areas of weakness and improve their performance
- providing a clear picture of individual qualities and skills.

Most schools using tutor assessment report significant improvement in students' performance and input to the PBL tutorials after receiving feedback from their tutor. But there may be times when the report has adverse effects on the relationship between the tutor and student. The main disadvantages of this type of assessment are:

- Students may believe that the assessment does not reflect their actual performance in PBL tutorials.
- Tutors can find it difficult to address the criteria and the rating scales provided in the report.
- Students' performance and input can vary, making it difficult for the tutor to translate their observations into an objective report.
- Tutors vary in the way they rank students. They may ignore the extremes of the scale and rank near the centre of the scale. Some may give students a higher ranking than is appropriate while others may underestimate the work of their students and give a lower ranking.

However, schools using this type of assessment are aware of these challenges and use evaluation and monitoring techniques to ensure standardisation of the process.

GETTING THE BEST FROM TUTOR ASSESSMENT

Your questions at this stage should be, 'If this type of assessment is used in my school, how can I get the best from it?' 'What should I do to ensure the best outcomes?'

First, understand each criterion in the report.

Second, think about problem-solving skills, self-directed learning, communication and personal skills, contribution to teamwork, commitment and medical knowledge and any other competencies highlighted by your school.

Third, identify your strengths and weaknesses and what you need to do to improve your performance in areas of deficiency. You might include in your plan: (1) learning support provided by your school, (2) how you will acquire these skills, (3) how you will evaluate your progress, and (4) how you will use feedback from your tutor to improve your performance.

Fourth, during your meeting with your tutor, discuss the limitations and negotiate any suggestions to help you improve.

Fifth, change your self-directed learning approach to suit the needs of the new course and the style of the PBL assessment.

And finally, monitor your progress and your contribution to the PBL tutorials, record your progress and take into account the criteria highlighted in the report (see Table 10.2).

GETTING THE MOST OUT OF FEEDBACK SESSIONS
TIP 1 COME WITH A POSITIVE ATTITUDE

If you come to the meeting with a firm belief that feedback is essential to your growth, you will benefit from the session. You can use the following strategies to maintain your positive thoughts about the meeting:

- Focus on how the meeting with your tutor could help you identify skills you should improve.

TABLE 10.2 Monitoring your progress

Competence	Related skills	Your areas of strength	Skills you are working on
Communication and interpersonal skills	Demonstrating good listening skills		
	Clarifying issues discussed		
	Asking open-ended questions that can help the group discussion		
	Showing respect to the views of other members in the group		
	Adding to what has already been discussed and thinking laterally		
	Targeting deep understanding		
	Being passionate about working with others		
Problem-solving skills	Identifying problems		
	Generating hypotheses		
	Collecting information		
	Employing reasoning process		
	Interpreting clinical and laboratory findings		
	Making priorities between hypotheses		
	Designing management plans		
Self-directed learning skills	Designing and implementing a satisfactory learning strategy to rectify deficiency in knowledge		
	Monitoring the adequacy of personal knowledge and skills		
	Identifying learning resources needed		
	Assessing effectiveness and efficiency of self-directed strategies		
Contribution to teamwork	Interacting with other members in an appropriate and effective way		
	Contributing to constructive and critical examination of issues discussed		
	Giving and receiving constructive feedback that enhances group function, improves performance and enforces shared responsibilities		
	Recognising that quality of contribution makes a difference		

		Your areas of strength	Skills you are working on
TABLE 10.2 Monitoring your progress *continued*			
Competence	**Related skills**		
Medical knowledge	Formulating, organising, and articulating the basic knowledge that can explain the problem and help to understand it		
Commitment	Demonstrating the following qualities in the PBL tutorials: — interest in issues discussed — enthusiasm — punctuality — preparation — responsibility — motivation		

- Do not try to deny or defend yourself.
- Think about the value of achieving these skills.
- Consider the meeting as an opportunity for your success.
- Watch your body language

TIP 2 LISTEN CAREFULLY

Preparing yourself before the meeting will help you listen to your tutor and think about their feedback. Listening is an indication of maturity and willingness to improve your performance. The signs of poor listening skills are:
- failing to allow others the opportunity to speak
- not making proper eye contact with the speaker
- not paying attention to the speaker and interrupting
- ignoring what is discussed and focusing on your own views
- asking questions that show you are not listening
- demonstrating through your body language that you are not listening.

But you do need to avoid 'overdoing' the listening by:
- spending too much time listening
- not responding adequately to questions raised
- failing to express your views.

TIP 3 ASK QUESTIONS THAT WILL HELP

Six rules to follow when asking questions during a feedback interview:
- Show interest in what was discussed with you. Ask questions that build on your tutor's feedback and points discussed.
- Ask if there is anything in particular that could help you improve your skills.
- Keep your discussion short. Ask two or three key follow-up questions and then plan with your tutor what you need to do.
- Ask about the academic support available in your university.
- Ask about a follow-up meeting 2 or 3 weeks later to discuss your progress.
- Thank your tutor for the feedback and the chance to improve your skills.

TIP 4 MAKE THE RIGHT CHOICES

According to William Glasser, an international authority in the field of internal control psychology, what makes a difference in any situation are the choices we make. The powerful genetic instructions that are built into our genetic code drive our behaviour and the choices we make. The outside environment, including rewards and punishment, only provides us with information. It does not make us do anything. For example, when faced with exactly the same situation people differ in the way they behave and make decisions. Thus students who work in a system of rewards and punishment over an extended period can see themselves as 'out of control'. For them success or failure is directly related to forces outside themselves.

We are born with needs that we are genetically instructed to satisfy and our behaviour reflects our best attempts to satisfy these needs. However, we do have choices. Turn to your internal control; do not allow yourself to be pressured by external factors. We feel in control when we:

- make the right decisions
- observe our attitude and choose to convey the right one
- look at issues from different perspectives
- accept responsibility for our actions
- focus on values led by our dreams, not pushed by problems or situations.

TIP 5 PLAN WITH YOUR TUTOR

Do not be distracted by negative feedback from your tutor. Feedback is a great opportunity for all of us to improve our performance and reach our potential. Success lies on the far side of failure. The lesson here is: practise confronting your fears before they control your life. Start working on issues raised in the feedback sessions without delay:

- discuss your priorities
- identify skills and competencies you need to develop
- define areas that need further work
- establish a timeframe for your plan
- discuss resources and university support systems that can help you.

TIP 6 WORK ON YOUR PLAN IMMEDIATELY

Imagine that you are guaranteed success and achievement if you develop these skills and competencies by the end of the semester. Now think about these questions as you put your plan into action:

- What changes would I make now?
- What goals would I set if I were guaranteed success?
- What are my fears? Focus on a specific fear in your life. For example, scribing for the group, or debating an issue in the PBL tutorials. Your fears may be holding you back from realising your full potential.
- Whatever the answers to these questions, begin working today as though your success was guaranteed.

TIP 7 FOCUS ON COMPETENCIES

Developing a competence takes time. It is not a rapid fix to a problem. But you need to plan what you will achieve over a particular period to reach your potential. Your plan can be structured to allow you to work on your priorities on a daily basis. Think about these questions:

- What portion of each day have you set aside to develop this competence and practise the new skills?
- Have you considered both short- and long-term goals to develop these skills?
- Have you correctly identified the priority tasks to work on?

TIP 8 MONITOR YOUR PROGRESS

The aims of your monitoring process are to:

- ensure you are following your plan and committing the time allocated to each component
- ensure you are passionate about your work
- introduce self-motivation techniques to keep you focused
- record your progress and critically analyse your reflections
- identify new learning needs and objectives.

CONCLUSIONS

Assessment in a PBL curriculum targets competencies and skills including cognitive skills, application of knowledge, professionalism, communication skills and system-based practices. A number of tools are used in assessment including: multiple-choice questions, extended-matching questions, PBL-style questions, short-answer questions, portfolios, tutor assessment, student logbooks, and the objective structured clinical examination. Tutor assessment usually consists of standardised reports completed by the tutor and the tutor's feedback for each student. Such assessment is particularly useful because areas that cannot be examined by conventional methods can be assessed, for example, listening skills and interaction with other members in the group, personal attributes, dealing with uncertainties and handling challenging situations, contributing to group dynamics and group success and demonstrating professional values such as reliability and integrity. The tips provided will help you get the best from the feedback session with your tutor.

FURTHER READING
BOOKS
Azer SA. Core clinical cases in basic biomedical science. London: Hodder–Arnold; 2006.
Coales U. PLAB 1000 extended-matching questions. London: The Royal Society of Medicine Press; 2000.
Feather A, Domizio P, Field BCT, et al. EMQs for medical students. Volumes 1, 2 & 3. PasTest; 2002.
Harden RM, Gleeson FA. Assessment of medical competence using an objective structured clinical examination (OSCE). Medical education booklet, No. 8. Edinburgh: Association for the Study of Medical Education; 1999.

Leung WC. MCQs in integrated sciences for medical students. Edinburgh: Churchill-Livingstone, 1999.

Seifert T, Harms S. Case files biochemistry. New York: Lange; 2005.

Toy EC, DeBord CRS, Wanger A, et al. Case files microbiology. New York: Lange; 2005.

Toy EC, Rosenfeld GC, Loose DS, et al. Case files pharmacology. New York: Lange; 2005.

Toy EC, Ross LM, Cleary LJ, et al. Case files gross anatomy. New York: Lange; 2005.

Toy EC, Weisbrodt NW, Dubinsky WP, et al. Case files physiology. New York: Lange; 2005.

ARTICLES AND RESEARCH PAPERS

Beullens J, Struyf E, Van Damme B. Do extended matching multiple-choice questions measure clinical reasoning? Med Educ 2005; 39(4):410–417.

Beullens J, Van Damme B, Jaspaert H, et al. Are extended-matching multiple-choice items appropriate for a final test in medical education? Med Teach 2002; 24(4):390–395.

Beullens J, Struyf E, Van Damme B. Diagnostic ability in relation to clinical seminars and extended-matching questions examinations. Med Educ 2006; 40(12):1173–1179.

Davis DA, Mazmanian PE, Fordis M, et al. Accuracy of physician self-assessment compared with observed measures of competence: a systematic review. JAMA 2006; 296(9): 1094–1102.

Eva KW, Reiter HI, Rosenfeld J, et al. The ability of the multiple mini-interview to predict preclerkship performance in medical school. Acad Med 2004; 79(10 Suppl):S40–S42.

Iramaneerat C, Yudkowsky R, Myford CM, et al. Quality control of an OSCE using generalizability theory and many-faceted Rasch measurement. Adv Health Sci Theory Pract 2007; 20 Feb; [Epub ahead of print].

Kogan JR, Bellini LM, Shea JA. Feasibility, reliability, and validity and the mini-clinical evaluation exercise (mini-CEX) in a medicine core clerkship. Acad Med 2003; 78(Suppl 10):S33–S35.

Ladak A, Hanson J, de Gara CJ. What procedures are student doing during undergraduate surgical clerkship? Can J Surg 2006; 49(5):329–334.

McManus IC, Smithers E, Partridge P, et al. A levels and intelligence as predictors of medical careers in UK doctors: 20 years prospective study. BMJ 2003; 327(7407):139–142.

Norcini JJ. The mini clinical evaluation exercise (mini-CEX). Clin Teach 2005; 2(1):25–30.

Norcini JJ, Blank LL, Duffy FD, et al. The mini-CEX: a method for assessing clinical skills. Ann Intern Med 2003; 138(6):478–810.

Reiter HI, Eva KW, Hatala RM, et al. Self and peer assessment in tutorials: application of a relative-ranking model. Acad Med 2002; 77(11):1134–1139.

Rushton A. Formative assessment: a key to deep learning. Med Teach 2005; 27(6):509–513.

CHAPTER 11

Keys for examination success

Destiny is not a matter of chance, it is a matter of choice; it is not a thing to be waited for, it is a thing to be achieved.

WILLIAM JENNINGS BRYAN

INTRODUCTION

When I was a medical student some time ago, one of my friends said, 'Examinations are like a gift box. You never know what you're going to get'. For several years I believed her; I even quoted it at times when as a student I shared my views about examinations. But years later, when I had I learnt about medical education and became an examiner, question writer, curriculum designer—and a student again—I no longer believed my friend's statement. Examinations should not be a surprise. Good students can identify over 80 per cent of the questions. They have developed the ability and intuition to identify key issues in what they learn, focus on competencies highlighted in the curriculum and critically reflect on concepts raised that can be of clinical significance.

This chapter will change your views about examinations and provide you with the secrets for success in examination. Mastering the keys and putting them into practice will help you improve your final scores. I list the main pitfalls students encounter at examination and give you the secrets to think like an examiner—to prepare for your examinations with a new perspective.

PREPARATION FOR EXAMINATION

Simply reading your textbooks and classroom notes will not improve your ability to answer questions. To prepare for your examination you need to rehearse what you will be doing during the test. For example:
* organising information to justify a particular hypothesis
* constructing a flow chart to show underlying mechanisms and pathogenesis of patient's presenting symptoms
* searching for new information by asking questions that can delineate priorities among your hypotheses and exclude some.

The aim of your revision is to duplicate the conditions you will be facing in the examination. These will differ depending on the format and objectives of the examination. For example, in a clinical examination such as an objective structured clinical examination (OSCE), which consists of a series of timed stations, each one focused on a particular task, you may be asked to undertake a specific task which could include: (1) interviewing the patient and taking a medical history, (2) examining the patient and eliciting clinical signs, (3) presenting a summary of the medical history, clinical findings and your differential diagnosis, and (4) responding to the examiners' questions in regard to clinical findings, diagnosis, laboratory investigations needed and the overall management plan.

Thus your preparation should focus on strategic learning.

- Collect information about the examination you are going to undertake, what you need to do, the duration of the test, and the challenges you might face in your examination.
- Spend more time thinking about information learnt and how you can apply it to solve problems than reading textbooks and reviewing papers.
- Use previous examinations to learn about the tasks you will be doing in the examination and the style of questions.
- Review your problem-based learning (PBL) cases, learning notes and summary sheets.

Preparation for your examinations is vital for your success. The following steps will help you to organise your 'rehearsal'.

STEP 1 COLLECT INFORMATION

If you know the challenges you will face in the examination, you can focus your study efforts and sharpen your skills to address them. The challenges might include:

- overall structure of the examination
- educational principles behind the examination
- types of questions that will be asked
- kinds of answers your examiners expect from you
- material to be covered, the number of questions and the time to be spent on each question
- contribution of each examination to the overall mark
- attitudes, skills and professional competencies to be tested.

Do not leave finding answers to these challenges till the last minute of your preparation. Find the answers early in the semester. There are also a number of specific questions that you need to answer:

- Are the questions focused on PBL tutorials, lectures, seminars, or textbooks?
- What skills does the examination cover?
- Will the examination cover themes discussed in previous years as well?
- Are the questions focused on one discipline or integrated across disciplines?
- What types of question will be included—essay, multiple-choice, extended-matching, modified-essay, PBL-style?
- Are all questions to be answered or can you choose between questions?
- Will the questions be similar in their structure to last year's examination? If different, in what ways are they different?
- How many questions will be in the examination paper? How many hours are allowed for the examination? Is any time allowed for reading?

You might find answers to these questions by:

- searching for information in your subject guide or on the faculty website
- attending a review session on summative examinations
- reviewing past years' examinations
- asking the course coordinators or your PBL tutor
- asking students who have already taken these examinations.

STEP 2 THINK ABOUT KEY CONCEPTS COVERED

Your preparation for the examination should focus on:
- key concepts and learning objectives covered during the semester
- PBL cases (problems), key lectures, practical class resources and your summary sheets (Table 11.1 shows a template that you can use for summarising learning objectives)
- your action plan—prepared in light of the knowledge you have collected about the examination structure.

TABLE 11.1 Key learning objectives template

Week	PBL cases (problems)	Lectures	Practical classes	Multimedia/ other resources	Comments
1					
2					
3					
4					
5					
6					
7					
8					
9					
10					
11					
12					
13					
14					
15					

- Write down key learning objectives for each week.
- Think about the relationships between the learning objectives for 2 or 3 weeks. Think laterally to find the big picture. For example, shortness of breath may be discussed in some of the cardiovascular problems and then again in some of the respiratory problems: try to expand these relationships and identify other causes.
- Develop a strategic plan for your revision work.

STEP 3 STUDY PAST EXAMINATIONS

By answering questions from past examinations, you will be able to:
- target important concepts and themes raised in the semester
- practise the application of knowledge learnt and test your understanding

- test your ability to integrate knowledge, generate hypotheses, make priorities and solve problems
- mentally prepare yourself for examination tasks
- practise managing your anxiety and maximising your ability to use examination time effectively.

STEP 4 REVIEW YOUR LEARNING RESOURCES

The learning resources you need for your preparation may include:
- PBL cases (problems)
- your group's notes and summaries of learning issues
- your own learning summary sheets, flow charts, mechanisms, summary tables and diagrams
- lecture notes, seminars and PowerPoints
- online review questions (most schools have developed their online bank of questions)
- review textbooks that integrate concepts and discuss PBL cases and supplement what you have learnt in your course
- anatomy atlas and your anatomy diagrams (keep your subject textbooks for reference when you need to check a specific issue).

How do you use these learning resources in your review?
- Be sure that you understand the key principles behind what you are reviewing.
- Use diagrams and flow charts to organise key information and visualise important processes.
- Link fine detail from lectures and textbooks to learning concepts raised in the PBL cases. This allows you to explore relationships between disciplines and study the interaction between basic and clinical sciences.
- Do not try to review each PBL case on its own: think about relationships between two or three cases you have studied in your course, identify relationships and their significance. For example, haematemesis (vomiting blood) as a learning issue could be identified in a problem covering peptic ulcer and then in another problem on liver cirrhosis and oesophageal varices. Ask yourself, what are the main differences between the two problems? What else could produce haematemesis? What are the management goals of each problem?
- Link your review process with the learning objectives you have identified. Ask yourself how the information you are reviewing could be applied to address questions in the examination.
- By reviewing a body system, you can establish relationships between disciplines such as anatomy, histology, physiology, pathophysiology, microbiology and the patient's signs and symptoms. This approach is reinforced by using PBL cases.

STEP 5 PREPARE FOR EXAMINATION CONDITIONS

Each examination has its own challenges. Table 11.2 summarises the skills covered in the examination and what you need to do in your preparation.

TABLE 11.2 Skills required for assessment and your preparation

Assessment	Skills covered	Preparation needed
Written examination (scenario-based MCQs)	Ability to: — answer a large number of questions that encompass core components of the curriculum — understand the case scenario, the stem and the distractors and think laterally for relationships — interpret cues in the scenario, exclude less likely items and choose the most likely item on the basis of supportive evidence available	Interpreting cues provided in a case scenario Understanding the question Lateral thinking Weighing evidence for and against the distractors provided Completing answers within the time allocated Answering all components of the question Practising similar questions under exam conditions
Clinical examination (e.g. OSCE)	Clinical competency broken down into various components (e.g. taking a history, examining the abdomen, interpreting an X-ray) Ability to: — complete a task at each station within a specified time — demonstrate communication and interpersonal skills — demonstrate procedural skills	Communication and interpersonal skills Understanding the question Targeting key issues and making priorities Procedural skills Collection of evidence and weighing it for and against different hypotheses Completing answers within the time allocated
PBL-style questions	Ability to: — generate hypotheses — design an enquiry plan — interpret clinical findings and investigation results — weigh the evidence for and against an hypothesis — provide justification — build a mechanism showing pathogenesis of a disease — make decisions and handle uncertainty — design a management plan	Interpreting cues provided in the case scenario Lateral thinking Mastering the cognitive skills addressed in the questions Changing learning strategies to address these needs Completing answers within the time allocated Practising similar questions under exam conditions

TOP 10 PITFALLS OF EXAMINATIONS
PITFALL 1 NOT ANSWERING THE QUESTION

Problem: This is a very common problem: students do not address the keywords in the stem of the question. This may be the result of:
- failing to carefully read the question
- not understanding what exactly is needed
- rushing to answer the question without planning

- not interpreting the cues in the stem of the question
- not doing enough preparation.

Tips: Reading the stem of the question more than one time is recommended. Underline keywords in the stem and ask yourself questions such as: 'What is the significance of these keywords?' 'Do I understand the question?' 'What exactly is this question about?' 'What are the subheadings I need to include in my answer?' 'How much time should I spend on the question?' 'Is this question about breadth or depth of knowledge or both?' 'Do I need to compare, justify, or present an argument?' 'What strategies should I use to present my answers: should I use a diagram, then text, or a table or flow chart?' 'How will a table help?' 'If I decide to use a table what headings do I need to construct?'

Questions like these will help you understand the question and organise and present your answers correctly.

PITFALL 2 FAILING TO ANSWER PART OF THE QUESTION

Problem: Many examiners would agree that this is another common pitfall. Students often spend a lot of time answering only one component of a question. This is not necessarily due to a lack of knowledge, but more likely a failure to recognise each item in the question or rushing to answer the question without giving it enough thought.

Tips: Before starting your answer, check how many components the question has and how much time you need to spend on each. In addition to underlining each component, develop the habit of rereading the stem before moving to the next question.

PITFALL 3 SPENDING TOO MUCH TIME ANSWERING ONE QUESTION

Problem: Students who do not prepare for their examinations usually fall into this trap. They spend a lot of time answering the first few questions and end up not having enough time to answer the last questions. In most cases they miss out, not because they do not know the answer but because they do not know how to organise their time.

Tips: Part of the preparation process is to know how many questions you will face in your examination, the type of questions and the total time allocated for the examination. Preparation also includes practising answering similar questions under examination conditions, learning how to deal with stress during examinations and how to plan your answers and complete your responses within the time allowed. The number of marks allocated for each question, if provided, can be very helpful: you will spend more time on a question worth 15 marks than on a question worth 5 marks.

PITFALL 4 NOT ORGANISING ANSWERS

Problem: Lack of organisation in answers can take a number of forms:
- not using headings and subheadings
- starting with less important issues

- not demonstrating consistency in the argument
- not presenting a logical flow in the argument
- not writing legibly
- lacking focus; not targeting key principles
- not keeping each answer in one place; writing notes to the examiner such as 'see the last page' or 'other answers are on the back of this page' or 'ignore answers in black'.

Tips: Consider the key issues of the question and the best way to present your answers. Before you start, write the outline of your answer in pencil. Think about how your answer will progress and the space you will use.

Organising your answers will have a major impact on the examiner. It allows them to follow your argument, allocate marks to each part you have addressed, identify keywords and terms you have used and assess your justification, reasoning or interpretation of findings.

PITFALL 5 NOT COVERING THE BREADTH AND DEPTH NEEDED

Problem: This pitfall is related to the first two pitfalls: students do not understand if the question is about the breadth or depth of knowledge, or both. They do not realise the significance of keywords in the stem such as: 'list', 'write a brief summary', 'justify', 'provide evidence', 'list and provide examples for each item', 'discuss', 'explain', 'provide a flow chart showing', 'draw a diagram showing the mechanism'. For example, when the examiner asks you to present a list, they are looking for the breadth of your knowledge in this area. On the other hand, when they ask you to make a list and provide examples or a justification for each item, the question is targeting the breadth and depth of knowledge.

Tips: Understanding what is needed and the keywords in the question are vital. Preparation for this element of the examination will foster your skills. Ask your tutor to give you feedback on your answers and your approach in handling previous years' papers. Do not waste time on issues unrelated to the question or which are insignificant and will not form the bulk of the answer.

PITFALL 6 NOT LABELLING DIAGRAMS

Problem: Including a diagram in your answers without labelling its different parts will be a waste of time and will not add marks to your answer even if the diagram is correct. Diagrams demonstrate your understanding of the different components of a structure, organ, or body system, their names and information regarding different components. Labelling is vital and should be clearly and correctly done.

Tips: As part of your examination preparation, practise drawing and labelling diagrams. Labelling diagrams usually consists of two components: major structures and fine details. Give equal attention to both.

PITFALL 7 BECOMING STRESSED

Problem: Stress during examinations may be the result of a number of factors:
- not using correct preparation strategies or not doing enough preparation
- coming late to the examination

- not sleeping well the night before
- spending a lot of time on difficult questions
- not organising answers or planning the time needed for each question
- coming to the examination with negative thoughts
- dealing with personal problems (e.g. finances); not focused on the course.

Tips: Stress during examinations can be avoided or minimised. Work on the causes of the stress to help minimise it.

PITFALL 8 NOT BEING STRATEGIC

Problem: Students fail to be strategic in their answers when they:
- focus on trivia and ignore major concepts
- present their answers in a hesitant way; are unable to make clear decisions
- do not use appropriate language
- do not demonstrate a logical flow
- do not target the focus of the question
- do not use appropriate tools (e.g. tables, flow charts)
- include redundant statements
- include incorrect statements
- do not demonstrate understanding of the educational principles behind the question
- do not engage the examiner or present a strong case
- fail to plan their answers.

Tips: Think about ways to maximise your marks. Spend time rehearsing before examinations.

PITFALL 9 NOT USING APPROPRIATE SCIENTIFIC OR MEDICAL TERMS

Problem: Examiners are usually looking for keywords in your answers. For example, if the question is about the pathogenesis of bronchial asthma, you might need to include in your answers keywords such as: 'atopy', 'allergy', 'bronchospasm', 'occupational sensitiser', 'atmospheric pollution', 'genetic factors', 'airway hyperresponsiveness', 'inflammatory mediators', 'vascular leakage', 'allergens'.

Tips: Effective use of medical and scientific terms related to the question is important. Examiners search for keywords as they allocate marks.

PITFALL 10 NOT TURNING UP OR TURNING UP TO THE WRONG PLACE

Problem: This problem is usually the result of poor organisational skills: not reading the examination schedule carefully enough, confusing the examination venue with other places in the university, failing to check a map or coming late to the examination.

Tips: Use a map to identify the examination venue. If you have never been there, visit the venue the day before the examination and plan to be there at least half an hour before the start of the examination.

THINK LIKE AN EXAMINER

How does the examiner plan for examinations? This might look like a strange question. Why do you need to know about strategies used by the examiner? How will this knowledge help you?

Remember there are two players in assessment: you (the examinee) and the examiner (assessment designer). Each player has a target to work towards: you are working towards passing this hurdle (the examination) and the examiner is working to construct an examination that allows the faculty to evaluate whether you have learnt the skills, competencies and attitudes targeted in the curriculum. So how do examiners prepare examinations?

Table 11.3 is a comparison of the two approaches and allows us to examine whether they match and it demonstrates a significant difference between what students and assessment designers do to prepare for examinations.

Students start with a collection of information about examinations, their structure, the style of questions, total number of questions, and previous examinations but they usually ignore the learning objectives, competencies and skills highlighted in the curriculum and the educational values behind the assessment.

Students want to remember information, lists, and mnemonics related to the content, but fail to focus on the key principles and themes addressed in the curriculum. They do not ask themselves questions like: 'What are the main concepts and principles covered in the semester?', 'What are the learning objectives of the contents covered?', 'If I am the examiner, what issues would I include in the examination?', 'What were the learning objectives covered in previous examinations?', 'How will the examiner turn the learning objectives into questions?', 'What new questions could be created to add to these questions?', 'Are there any other concepts that are related to these questions?'

COMPETENCIES, SKILLS AND ASSESSMENT TOOLS

The current trend in assessment is to design it so that competencies and skills identified in the curriculum, rather than specific topics or knowledge, are tested. To do this, appropriate assessment tools must be used. For example, to assess the ability of students to retrieve knowledge, examiners could use multiple-choice questions and short-answer questions, while to assess their ability to select and use information to solve problems, examiners could use modified essay questions and PBL-style questions.

Table 11.4 is based on George Miller's conceptual pyramid for clinical competence (Fig 11.1) and provides information about competencies to be tested, the skills related to each competency and the appropriate assessment tools that can be used to test these skills.

THINK LIKE AN EXAMINER: FINAL WORDS

Pay attention to how the examiners plan for examinations. You need to examine the learning objectives covered in PBL cases, lectures, and any other material covered during the course. You also need to think about competencies, skills, and key knowledge and

TABLE 11.3 How examiners and examinees prepare for examinations

Examiners (assessment designers)	Examinees (students)
1. Learning objectives Examiners usually start by mapping the learning objectives of PBL cases, lectures, practical classes and any other material used in the curriculum.	*1. Collection of information* Students usually start by collecting information about the examination such as: 'What type of examination is it?', 'How does the examination contribute to the total mark?', 'What type of questions?', 'Will we need to write chemical equations or chemical formulas in biochemistry?'
2. Competencies, skills and attitudes Examiners group these learning objectives under assessment categories such as competencies, skills, attitudes as per the structure of the curriculum used in the faculty.	*2. Goal setting and planning* The information gained highlights what is likely to be in the examination and helps students focus their learning processes, plan their review process and subsequent preparation for examinations. For example, if the examination questions focus on memorisation of factual knowledge, in their learning students will target lists, mnemonics and memorisation for recall. If the questions focus on understanding of subject matter, solving problems, analysing findings, generating hypotheses or providing supportive evidence, students will use a different learning approach.
3. Assessment tools Examiners have identified the tools to be used in assessing these competencies and skills. These tools may be MCQs, EMQs, short-answer questions, PBL-style questions or OSCE. They also examine the validity and the reliability of assessment tools used (see Glossary). How could these tools be used to match the philosophy of the curriculum?	*3. Practising past examinations* Most students like to see past examinations and work out the answers. This orients them to the style of questions they will face in the examination.
4. Writing questions At this stage examiners create questions that reflect the learning objectives, competencies, skills and attitudes highlighted in the curriculum. They use several tools to ensure that these skills and competencies are examined in different circumstances.	*4. Reviewing what they studied* Most students think that reading as much as they can of the material taught helps them prepare for examinations.
5. Evaluation of the questions Statistical analysis of the questions and feedback from students help improve the quality of examinations for the next year. This does not mean using the same questions, just the learning objectives addressed in previous examinations.	*5. Asking past students* If the faculty does not release previous examinations some students try to discover the topics covered by asking students from earlier years. This process will not help; you might even receive the wrong information.

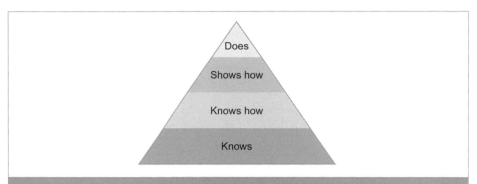

FIGURE 11.1 Miller's conceptual pyramid for clinical competence.

TABLE 11.4 A blueprint for assessment: competencies, skills and appropriate assessment tools		
Competencies	**Skills**	**Assessment tools**
Knows: To assess the ability of students to retrieve factual knowledge	Understanding concepts Understanding related fine details Integration of knowledge Justification and reasoning skills Categorisation of information	Multiple-choice questions Extended-matching questions Short-answer questions
Knows how: To assess the ability of students to use and apply information learnt to solve problems	Generating hypotheses Integration of information Clinical judgement skills Data gathering skills Analytical skills Using 'forward' and 'backward' reasoning Designing a management plan	Modified-essay questions PBL-style questions
Shows how: To assess the ability of students to use knowledge and skills in a controlled setting	History taking Clinical examination skills Procedural skills Data gathering skills Application of knowledge and problem-solving skills	Computer-based simulated exercise Practical laboratory stations Triple-jump examination OSCE Standardised patients
Does: Assesses the ability of students to use knowledge and skills in everyday challenges	Communication and interpersonal skills Setting priorities Professional relationships Clinical skills Interpretation skills Data gathering skills Decision-making skills Evaluation skills	Direct observation Peer assessment Preceptor rating scale Mini-clinical evaluation exercise Patient rating 360-degree evaluation (see Ch 12)

attitudes highlighted in the curriculum. Then ask yourself how the different assessment tools used by your faculty assess these competencies and skills. Think about the key learning objectives covered in past examinations and how the different assessment tools were used. By reviewing and preparing for your examinations with the same strategies used by the examiners you will be more focused in your learning and in targeting the competencies, attitudes and key knowledge you have to master.

24 KEYS FOR EXAMINATION SUCCESS

> Good judgement comes from experience, and often experience comes from bad judgement.
> RITA MAE BROWN

Success in examinations is not simply based on how many hours you spent learning; it is related to the quality of your preparation and the skills you worked on and highlighted in your preparation. The following keys will help you focus your preparation to target success.

→ KEY 1 REVIEW WITH AN EXAMINATION-ORIENTED APPROACH

When reading the material you studied, focus on the key principles behind it. Think about how this information could be a topic in your examination and how it could be used in answering a question. Study with a critical mind to find answers to questions such as: 'What is the justification available so far?', 'What is the underlying mechanism?', 'How are these issues related to what I already know?', 'What are my conclusions?' The more you are engaged in your review and focused on similar questions, the more you are preparing yourself and visualising how to use information learnt for the purpose of the examination.

→ KEY 2 MANAGE YOUR PREPARATION TIME

Time management is vital not just for your examination preparation but also as a habit you need to develop for your long-term success. Train yourself to focus for an allocated time and work effectively to achieve specific goals within a certain period of time to foster your skills, concentration span and prepare you for the examination situation. Do not try to learn new information in the last minutes before the examination.

→ KEY 3 VISUALISE YOUR SUCCESS

Switch your mind to positive mode. Develop the desire to achieve and score higher. Avoid thoughts that put you down or move you away from your target. Avoid phone calls, and visitors who distract you, upset you or disturb your preparation, particularly on the day of the examination or the night before.

→ KEY 4 STAY HEALTHY

Be aware of stress associated with examinations. It can increase the risk of becoming ill in the middle of your examinations. You can do many things to decrease that risk. By 3 weeks before the start of your examination you should be avoiding:
* changes in your study pattern, for example, all-night studying which will disturb your sleep cycle

- excessive intake of caffeine and other stimulants because they can increase your anxiety
- changing your eating pattern. Always practise healthy eating habits
- other stressful situations that may add to your stress, for example, working long days before examinations.

I also recommend that you use relaxation techniques, sleep sensibly, listen to music and seek social support from family and your friends. There is evidence from research that classical music stimulates areas of the brain responsible for creative thought and can enhance the process of coordination of information.

→ KEY 5 CHECK THE EXAMINATION TIMETABLE

Be sure that you have the final version of the examination timetable and have organised your revision timetable accordingly. Check the examination venue. If you have never been there, go and find out exactly where it is.

→ KEY 6 PREPARE YOURSELF

The day before an examination, get everything you need ready in a small container: your examination ID, pens, pencils, calculator with new batteries (if permitted), highlighter pens and an eraser. Go to bed earlier than usual. On the day of the examination, do not overload yourself with new information. Do not argue or discuss examination-related issues with anyone. Avoid doing anything that could increase your anxiety or stress. Aim to be at the examination venue about 30 minutes before the start. There is no harm in getting there early but it will be a great harm if you arrive late.

→ KEY 7 FOLLOW THE EXAMINATION RULES

Once you enter the examination room, follow these general rules:
- Ensure you are sitting at the desk assigned to you. Check the desk number.
- Listen carefully to the instructions given to you.
- Do not start before you are asked to.
- During the reading time, you should not touch your pencil or write anything. It is reading time.
- Do all administrative work you are asked to do such as candidate number, desk number, subject number, the date. Double check that you have written the correct information.
- Once you are in the examination room, do not talk to anyone.

→ KEY 8 USE READING TIME EFFECTIVELY

- Carefully check the instructions on the cover page of the examination paper.
- Check the marks allocated for each question.
- Check the number of questions you need to answer and whether there are compulsory questions.
- Work out the time needed to answer each question if this information was not given to you before the examination.
- Think about the components of each question you need to address.
- If you have choices, decide on the questions you are going to answer.
- Decide on the question you will start with.

➔ KEY 9 MANAGE EXAMINATION ANXIETY

One hundred years ago Yerkes and Dodson postulated a law about stress among students and its impact on learning. According to this law, people under low or high stress learn the least while those under moderate stress learn the most. There is a strong body of evidence from research to support this law. The lesson here is that you should learn how to use stress for your benefit.

There is evidence that people become less stressed during examinations when they:

- start preparing themselves to handle stressful situations when they commence their course
- replace negative thoughts with positive and encouraging ones
- use techniques such as meditation to overcome stress
- seek help if they cannot manage their own stress
- visualise their success and believe in their ability
- prepare for examinations and practise past examinations.

➔ KEY 10 UNDERLINE KEYWORDS IN THE QUESTION

Before rushing to answer a question, ensure that you understand the question. Ask yourself: 'What does this question mean?', 'What are the key issues I need to discuss in my answer?' The more you focus on keywords in the stem of the question the better your answer will be.

It is very important that you identify the 'instruction' words provided in the question. Commonly used instruction words include:

- Explain
- List
- Justify
- Give examples
- Differentiate between
- Provide evidence/reasons
- Construct/build a mechanism
- Discuss
- Describe
- Show
- Compare
- Evaluate

Identifying these instruction words is very important as these words can make a significant difference to the way you present your answer, for example, if you are asked to list the causes of shortness of breath versus if you are asked to justify why you think the patient's shortness of breath is due to pulmonary fibrosis versus if you are asked to build the mechanism underlying the patient's shortness of breath.

➔ KEY 11 ANSWER ALL OF THE QUESTION

Excessive stress might make you rush and forget to answer parts of a question. To avoid this, carefully read the question, put a number at the beginning of each part of the question, and when you complete your answers, check that you have covered each part.

→ KEY 12 DO NOT RUSH

If you are answering a short-answer question, do not rush to answer the question. Spend 1–2 minutes organising your thoughts. Write the main concepts to be covered in pencil as a checklist. Also write down the sub-items you will cover in your answer. Review the question again and check that you have covered everything asked in the question. Start answering the question, review your answer and edit as needed.

→ KEY 13 PLAN YOUR ANSWERS

The clearer you are about the keywords in the question stem and issues you need to address, the more you are able to decide on the best tool to use to present your answers. For example:

- A table is useful in comparing concepts and presenting different characteristics of each component. If you think that a table is the best way for you to present your answers, decide how many columns you need, what the headings will be and what items you will include in the table.
- A diagram is useful in showing different structures, relationships and possibly the function of each component/structure. Label it appropriately.
- A flow chart is useful in showing the sequence of events, cause/effect relationships, contributing factors and how the process has progressed.
- A box is useful in showing key points, causes, hypotheses and factors summarised as a list.

    Some questions may require you to use one or more of these tools to present your answers.

→ KEY 14 USE APPROPRIATE KEYWORDS

Every question triggers a number of keywords or scientific terms that you should use in your answer. Examiners will be looking for these keywords as they mark your paper. Successful students often do a brainstorming exercise and write down a list of the keywords related to the question. They also plan how to use these keywords under each sub-heading in their answer. The more you include related keywords in your answer, in an appropriate manner, the more marks you will gain.

→ KEY 15 DO NOT CONTRADICT YOURSELF

Sometimes, when students are not sure about what to say or what decision to make, they contradict themselves. Examiners will notice these contradictory statements, the student's struggle and their inability to present a concrete view. If you present contradictory statements in your answers, you will lose marks. Students who write contradictory statements are not necessarily unaware of the correct answers. In many cases, they did not read the question carefully, give themselves enough time to understand the question, weigh the evidence for and against each decision or organise their thoughts and they did not plan their answers.

→ KEY 16 BALANCE YOUR ANSWERS

Always ensure that your answers are well balanced and cover the big picture as well as the fine details. Some students either present a broad outline of the topic with no details, or only partly address the big picture and focus on a lot of unnecessary detail.

Neither approach is satisfactory. Successful students know how to address these two aspects in a balanced way.

→ KEY 17 TARGET THE HEART OF THE QUESTION

Many students spend a lot of time wandering around the question: they do not address the main issues, they do not target the heart of the question. If you want to write an introduction to your answer, write a very brief introduction, about one or two lines that lead you to the main issues raised in the question. If the question is about causes, reasons or hypotheses, start with important and related causes, then place less important causes at the end of your list.

Always think about ways you can show the examiner that you have understood the question. Present a clear, organised answer with no redundant sentences that demonstrates deep understanding, keeps to the point and shows you have no hesitation in writing your answer.

→ KEY 18 DO NOT OVER-INTERPRET YOUR FINDINGS

If you are asked to interpret clinical findings, laboratory or investigation results, do not try to over-interpret your findings. When you present your interpretation:
- Be sure that you understand the question.
- Always link your interpretation to the case scenario and any clinical findings.
- State common things first.
- Weigh the evidence for and against each interpretation. Assess any other supportive findings for your views.
- State other possibilities. Explain why these possibilities are less likely.
- Use lateral thinking in finding relationships.

→ KEY 19 IMPRESS THE EXAMINER

If you ask examiners what they need to see in an answer to maximise marks, most of them would say the answer will:
- answer the question asked
- be well organised
- be legibly written
- contain sentences that are complete—no telegraphic messages
- be as specific as possible
- include examples where needed
- demonstrate an understanding of the question
- be comprehensive: show an understanding of the subject
- contain no redundant information
- include justification for arguments.

These principles are universal and you should train yourself to consider them in your answers.

→ KEY 20 BE SPECIFIC

Examiners expect you to write clear answers and be specific when you make choices. For example, if the question is about what investigations you would order for the patient at this stage, many students may answer by stating, '(1) blood test, (2) X-ray, or (3) CT scan'. Such answers are not useful at all. Examiners expect you to be specific, for example by saying, '(1) Full blood examination and a blood film, (2) X-ray of the right forearm, or (3) CT scan of the cervical spine'.

→ KEY 21 AVOID TELEGRAPHIC MESSAGES

Some students write telegraphic messages. Their statements are not complete sentences and are not meaningful. Such answers confuse examiners and result in a loss of marks.

Successful students write sentences that:
*   have a clear purpose
*   contain no confusing words
*   clearly convey the answer without need for further detail
*   are meaningful and self-explanatory: the examiner does not have to reread them to understand what is meant
*   contain keywords and scientific terms related to the question
*   engage the reader: the sentences and paragraphs are thoughtfully woven and linked together
*   target the issues raised in the question.

→ KEY 22 EXPLAIN ABBREVIATIONS

As a general rule, in examinations you should never use abbreviations, even commonly used ones, unless you spell them out first—abbreviations can have several meanings. Also use correct units, for example 'mmHg' for blood pressure, '°C' for body temperature, and 'per minute' for pulse rate and respiratory rate.

→ KEY 23 MANAGE YOUR TIME WISELY

Some students spend too much time on one question, ending up with no time to answer one or more of the remaining questions. The following strategies will help you manage your time:
*   Adjust the time you spend on each question according to the allocated marks. For example, if the examination is for 2 hours and the total marks for the examination are 120 marks: 25 marks for Question 1, 15 marks for Question 2, 20 marks for Question 3, 20 marks for Question 4, 15 marks for Question 5, and 25 marks for Question 6, you might allocate your time as follows: 25 minutes for 1, 15 minutes for 2, 20 minutes for 3, 20 minutes for 4, 15 minutes for 5, and 25 minutes for 6.
*   Plan to complete your answers 2 minutes earlier than the allocated time; the extra time can be used towards the end to check your answers.
*   Managing your time during an examination is a skill that you need to practise before the examination.

→ KEY 24 CHECK THROUGH

Allow yourself the last 10–12 minutes of the examination time to run through your answers:
*   Ensure you have not missed any question or a part of a question.
*   Check the questions and your answers.
*   Underline your headings and subheadings.

CONCLUSIONS

Success in examinations requires a number of skills so you target the assessment objectives of your course. The top 10 pitfalls in examinations highlight the often small things that can make the difference between success and failure. Think like an examiner and turn your preparation from a student-based to an examiner-based preparation. Be clear about the objectives of each week, identify the competencies and the skills highlighted in the course and practise the examination situation you will face. Practise the 24 keys and you can improve your final marks dramatically.

FURTHER READING
BOOKS

Anderson LW, Krathwol D. A taxonomy for learning, teaching and assessment: a review of Bloom's taxonomy of educational objectives. New York: Longman; 2001.

Barnes R. Successful study for degrees. London: Routledge; 1995.

Girgis S, Hebert K, Burgess J. The insiders' guide to UK medical schools 2005/2006: The alternative prospectus compiled by the BMA medical students committee (illustrated). 8th edn. Oxford: Blackwell Publishing Ltd; 2005.

Race P. How to get a good degree. Buckingham: Open University; 1999.

Saks NS. How to excel in medical school. 3rd edn. Alexandria, Va: J&S Publishing; 2007.

ARTICLES AND RESEARCH PAPERS

Anderson J. Multiple choice questions revisited. Med Teach 2004; 26(2):110–113.

Azer SA. Assessment in a problem-based learning course. Twelve tips for constructing multiple choice questions that test students' cognitive skills. Biochem Molec Biol Educ 2003; 31(6):428–434.

Ben-David MF. The role of assessment in expanding professional horizons. Med Teach 2000; 22(5):472–477.

Fischer MR, Herrmann S, Kopp V. Answering multiple-choice questions in high-stakes medical examinations. Med Educ 2005; 39(9):890–894.

Holden NL. Multiple-choice questions: a guide to success. Br J Hosp Med 1993; 50(9): 557–559.

Lowry S. Assessment of students. BMJ 1993; 306 (6869):51–54.

Mavis BE. Does studying for an objective structured clinical examination a difference? Med Educ 2000; 34(10):808–812.

Miller GE. The assessment of clinical skills/competence/performance. Acad Med 1990; 65(9 Suppl):S63–S67.

Mires GJ, Ben-David MF, Preece PE, et al. Educational benefits of student self-marking of short-answer questions. Med Teach 2001; 23(5):462–466.

Moqattash S, Harris PF, Gumaa KA, et al. Assessment of basic medical sciences in an integrated systems-based curriculum. Clin Anat New York 1995; 8(2):139–147.

Palmer E, Devitt P. Constructing multiple choice questions as a method of learning. Ann Acad Med Singapore 2006; 35(9):604–608.

Schotanus JC. Student assessment and examination rules. Med Teach 1999; 21(3):318–321.

Seale KJ, Chapman J, Davey C. The influence of assessments on students' motivation to learn in a therapy degree course. Med Educ 2000; 34(8):614–621.

Smee S. ABC of learning and teaching in medicine: skill based assessment. BMJ 2003; 326(7391):703–706.

Sobral D T. What kind of motivation drives medical students' learning quest? Med Educ 2004; 38(9):950–957.

Yerkes RM, Dodson JD. The relation of strength of stimulus to rapidity of habit formation. J Comp Neurol Psychol 1908; 18:459482.

PART FOUR

THE SUCCESSFUL STUDENT IN PROBLEM-BASED LEARNING

CHAPTER 12

Non-cognitive skills and professionalism

Our profession is to heal. In a patient encounter, we consider a right and good healing action for that patient in his or her particular circumstances. A right healing action is one informed by the scientific and clinical evidence. A good action, in contrast, takes into account the patient's value and performances and is consistent with the physician's own clinical judgment.　　　　　**LYNNE KIRK**

INTRODUCTION

Although knowledge of medical sciences and competencies in reasoning, problem-solving and clinical medicine are essential to the making of a good doctor, patients may see things differently. Patients know that a doctor's ability to diagnose and manage their illnesses makes a big difference. Patients describe doctors as 'good' when they demonstrate up-to-date knowledge, excellent clinical skills, acceptable bedside manners, honesty and good moral and ethical standards. These are the basic attributes of professionalism and are applicable to all healthcare professions. Training medical and healthcare students in these competencies is a fundamental task of medical education.

Professionalism has become a universal component of undergraduate training in medical, nursing, physiotherapy, dentistry and other healthcare schools. Effective training in professionalism addresses a number of non-cognitive skills, humanistic attitudes and skills in moral reasoning as well as the effective use of interprofessional collaboration, communication in all aspects of the delivery of healthcare services and knowledge of the legal aspects of the profession. The focus is not only on the ethical dilemmas such as abortion, euthanasia, genetic testing and counselling highlighted in textbooks but also on the day-to-day moral, ethical and professional issues faced by junior doctors.

NON-COGNITIVE SKILLS

In current thinking on medical education, skills and competencies in the curriculum can be classified into two main groups:

1 *Cognitive skills*: generating hypotheses, designing an enquiry plan, researching for new information, weighing the evidence for and against hypotheses, performing procedures, using information technology, designing management plans, interpreting patient's laboratory and investigation results and making appropriate decisions.

2 *Non-cognitive skills or behaviours*: empathy, integrity, communication and interpersonal skills, responsibility, collaboration, cultural competence and continuous improvement (see Table 12.1).

TABLE 12.1 Examples of desirable non-cognitive values and their behaviours

Values/ qualities	Behaviours
Empathy	Demonstrates respectful behaviour when interacting with patients and their families Shows they are in charge of their attitude Is sensitive to the patient's needs
Integrity	Takes responsibility Keeps their word Maintains patient confidentiality Is not biased Creates and sustains ethically sound relationship with patients Places the interests of patients and society above their own Considers ethical and moral issues in their practice
Communication skills	Demonstrates good listening skills Is not sarcastic Is patient, not disruptive or hostile
Interpersonal skills	Works effectively with others Encourages and motivates people Has a positive attitude Knows how to serve other members in the team Opens the doors of opportunity to others Is gentle in their approach Focuses on patient satisfaction
Responsibility	Arrives on time Demonstrates a positive attitude Acknowledges their mistakes Focuses on outcomes
Collaboration	Builds bridges with others Shares information with others Focuses on people not just the task Feels happy when they work with others
Cultural competence	Respects people from other cultures Can build relationships with people from a range of backgrounds Is not judgemental Invests in their relationships with people from other cultures
Continuous improvement	Seeks to learn new skills Learns from their patients, peers, students, and supervisors Monitors their progress Plans their learning Learns from feedback

NON-COGNITIVE SKILLS: ESSENTIAL FOR SUCCESS

When you possess these skills you will:

- be respected; people will want to work with you and to seek your help
- be given opportunities to take leadership positions and influence others

- leave an excellent impression wherever you work
- be able to create a healthy and successful environment in your workplace.

WHAT IS PROFESSIONALISM?

Healthcare work is patient-centred. To be successful in your career you need to focus on the competencies emphasised by the profession, take good care of your patients and develop competencies in scientific and clinical medicine. Evidence from several publications shows that unsatisfactory performance is more likely to be the result of unprofessional behaviour or attitudes than the lack of scientific knowledge or clinical skills.

Professionalism is one of the main competencies you need to start developing during your undergraduate course. It will help you understand your duties and be able to reflect on your own performance. Professionalism comprises a set of values, behaviours, qualities and relationships that underpins the trust the public has in doctors and healthcare professionals. Values that form part of professionalism include:

- commitment to the moral and ethical values encouraged by the profession
- effective use of interprofessional collaboration and communication in all aspects of the delivery of healthcare services
- knowledge of legal aspects related to the profession
- non-cognitive values and behaviours as discussed above, for example, empathy, integrity, responsibility, interpersonal skills.

DEVELOPING PROFESSIONAL SKILLS

Developing these skills and qualities should be one of your targets. Do not focus on learning basic sciences, leaving professional skills to the clinical years. Problem-based learning emphasises these skills very early in the course. Work on these skills and take every opportunity you can to reflect on the values and qualities of professionalism. They need to become part of your habitual behaviour. Visualise them as your priorities and you will be effective in your approach. The following tips will help:

TIP 1 KNOW WHAT IS EXPECTED

The first step is understanding what are the qualities and behaviours for success. The better your understanding of these qualities and behaviours, the easier it is for you to acquire them. Some schools have policies that identify unacceptable behaviours and promote the good practices emphasised in the curriculum.

TIP 2 LEARN FROM ROLE MODELS

Role modelling is an integral component of medical and other healthcare curricula and is embedded at different stages of your undergraduate course. We identify people as role models when they inspire us, influence our work and motivate us to develop new skills and achieve our potential. One of the best ways to acquire at least some of the necessary non-cognitive skills is by observing how good teachers and professionals handle difficult situations, relate to their patients, deal with moral and ethical situations and work with their colleagues. These skills cannot be taught in lectures or seminars. We develop these skills by working closely with people who possess them. Invest time to work closely with good teachers who can be your role models.

A search of the MEDLINE and HighWire databases under 'good teacher', 'role model' and 'mentor' indicates that the subject of role modelling is attracting growing attention. From January 1978 to December 2003 the number of publications in English was 180, of which just over two-thirds appeared in the years 1999–2003 (Fig 12.1).

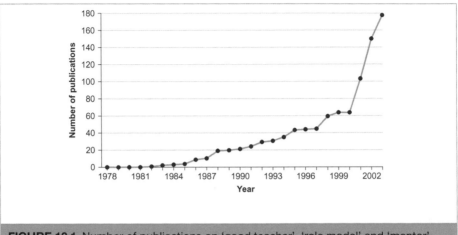

FIGURE 12.1 Number of publications on 'good teacher', 'role model' and 'mentor' (1978–2003).

TIP 3 REFLECT ON THE PARABLES YOU HEAR

In an excellent article by Stern and Papadakis, published in *The New England Journal of Medicine* (see Further reading), the authors argue that:

> Parables are a powerful means of transmission of cultural values; the norms of professional behaviour have been handed down through generations of doctors using stories with meaning. In medicine, parables often start with 'I had this great case' or 'when I was an intern'. What ensues is a story about a fascinating medical case with a moral about what it means to be a doctor. The published writing of William Carlos Williams, Jerome Groopman, Atul Grawande, and others take this process to its highest form. But these stories are exchanged every day in conversations over lunch, in the hallways and outside the hospital—a story about how a patient survived when perhaps he should not have, a story about how you would have missed the diagnosis had you not stopped to ask one more question, a story about an observation from a nurse that alerted you to an unexpected problem. These stories not only serve to transmit professional values but also reveal the struggle of how we try (and sometimes fail) to meet the highest standards of professional conduct. The tradition of story telling is instructive for students, but building it into a formal curriculum is a challenge.

Reflecting on these stories will help you learn:
- from the ethical and moral challenges behind the situations
- how to deal with uncertainty and difficult situations
- how to share your stories with your peers and ask for their views.

TIP 4 ASK FOR HELP

Most clinical schools build a learning culture and invest in student support services. To get the best out of these services you need first to identify what type of help you need then which of the services can help you. Effective use of student support services will help you to:
- develop new skills and competencies
- practise the use and implementation of skills learnt
- receive feedback on your performance from your teachers and peers
- work on specific tasks to achieve your goals
- receive support and encouragement as you progress
- feel good about yourself and your achievements.

TIP 5 LEARN FROM FEEDBACK

Many times we forget that formative assessment is an opportunity for us to learn and sharpen our objectives. As discussed in Ch 10, the aims of formative assessment are to guide future learning, provide reassurance, promote reflection and foster learning. The feedback that usually follows formative assessment targets students' behaviour and attributes and should give you opportunities to monitor your progress, work on areas of weakness and acquire new competencies and skills.

TIP 6 PRACTISE 360-DEGREE EVALUATION

360-degree evaluation is a mechanism for evaluating performance based on feedback from everyone the person comes in contact with, for example, peers, patients, nurses, clinicians, junior doctors, medical educators, other healthcare professionals. Because this evaluation comes from a wide range of people it can help you identify a wide range of skills you need to improve or develop.

TIP 7 IMPROVE YOUR ATTITUDE

When we are in charge of our attitude we can:
- improve our relationships with others
- exhibit desirable professional competencies and skills
- achieve our goals and reach our potential.

TIP 8 TURN THESE BEHAVIOURS INTO HABITS

Practise these behaviours daily and you will be able to turn them into habits that benefit you and the community you are serving. As part of this process:
- focus on changing your actions and habits, not the situation
- strive for the satisfaction of unselfish thinking
- monitor your progress
- focus on the outcomes you would like to achieve.

CONCLUSIONS

Non-cognitive skills are essential for your success. They also represent an important component of professionalism.

Professionalism will help you understand your duties and be able to reflect on your own performance. It comprises a set of values, behaviours, and relationships that underpins the trust the public has in doctors and healthcare professionals.

Successful medical and healthcare students start working on their non-cognitive skills very early in the course. This enables them to master these skills and turn them into habits that benefit themselves and the communities they serve.

FURTHER READING
BOOKS AND REPORTS

Accreditation Council for Graduate Medical Education. General competencies. Chicago: ACGME; 1999. Available: http://www.acgme.org/outcome/comp/comMin.asp; accessed 11 July, 2007.

Canadian Medical Association. Medical professionalism. A discussion paper on professionalism in medicine. CMA series of health care discussion papers. Available: http://www.cma.ca/index.cfm/ci_id/3300/la_id/1.htm; accessed 19 Feb, 2007.

The University of Western Ontario. Charter on medical/dental professionalism. Available: http://www.schulich.uwo.ca/Administration/Professionalism.pdf; accessed 19 Feb, 2007.

Makely S. Professionalism in health care: a primer for career success. 2nd edn. London: Pearson Higher Education; 2004.

Royal College of Physicians. Report of a working party. Doctors in society. Medical professionalism in a changing world. London: Royal College of Physicians; 2005. Available: http://www.rcplondon.ac.uk/pubs/books/docinsoc/docinsoc.pdf; accessed 19 Feb, 2007.

Schon DA. Educating the reflective practitioner: toward a new design for teaching and learning the professions. San Francisco: Jossey-Bass; 1987.

Stern DT. Measuring medical professionalism. Oxford: Oxford University Press; 2006.

ARTICLES AND RESEARCH PAPERS

American Board of Internal Medicine Foundation, American College of Physicians, American Society of Internal Medicine, European Federation of Internal Medicine. Medical professionalism in the new millennium: a physician charter. Ann Intern Med 2002; 136(3):243–246. Available: http://www.annals.org/cgi/reprint/136/3/243.pdf; accessed 19 Feb, 2007.

Blank L, Kimball H, McDonald W, et al. Medical professionalism in the new millennium. A physician charter 15 months later. Ann Intern Med 2002; 138(10):839–841.

Charon R. The patient–physician relationship. Narrative medicine: a model for empathy, reflection, profession and trust. JAMA 2001; 286(15):1897–1902.

Cruess RL, Cruess SR. Teaching professionalism: general principles. Med Teach 2006; 28(3):205–208.

Cruess SR, Cruess RL. Professionalism must be taught. BMJ 1997; 315(7123):1674–1677.

Fones CS, Kua EH, Goh LG. 'What makes a good doctor?' views of the medical profession and the public in setting priorities for medical education. Singapore Med J 1998; 39(12):537–542.

Gordon J. Progressing professionalism. Med Educ 2006; 40(10):936–938.

Higgs J. Physiotherapy, professionalism, and self-directed learning. J Sing Physio Assoc 1993; 14:8–11.

Leahy M, Cullen W, Bury G. "What makes a good doctor?" A cross sectional survey of public opinion. Ir Med J 2003; 96(2):38–41.
continued on p. 206

EVIDENCE-BASED LEARNING

Disciplinary action by medical boards and prior behavior in medical school

Evidence supporting professionalism as a critical measure of competence in medical education is limited. In a case-control study, the researchers investigated the association of disciplinary action against practicing physicians with prior unprofessional behavior in medical school. They also examined the specific types of behavior that are most predictive of disciplinary action against practicing physicians with unprofessional behavior in medical school.

The study included 235 graduates of three medical schools who were disciplined by one of 40 state medical boards between 1990 and 2003 (case physicians). The 469 control physicians were matched with the case physicians according to medical school and graduation year. Predictor variables from medical school included the presence or absence of narratives describing unprofessional behavior, grades, standardized-test scores, and demographic characteristics. Narratives were assigned an overall rating for unprofessional behavior. Those that met the threshold for unprofessional behavior were further classified among eight types of behavior and assigned a severity rating (moderate to severe).

The results show that disciplinary action by a medical board was strongly associated with prior unprofessional behavior in medical school (odds ratio, 3.0; 95 percent confidence interval, 1.9 to 4.8), for a population attributable risk of disciplinary action of 26 percent. The types of unprofessional behavior most strongly linked with disciplinary action were severe irresponsibility (odds ratio, 8.5; 95 percent confidence interval, 1.8 to 40.1) and severely diminished capacity for self-improvement (odds ratio, 3.1; 95 percent confidence interval, 1.2 to 8.2). Disciplinary action by a medical board was also associated with low scores on the Medical College Admission Test and poor grades in the first two years of medical school (1 percent and 7 percent population attributable risk, respectively), but the association with these variables was less strong than that with unprofessional behavior.

The researchers concluded that disciplinary action among practicing physicians by medical boards was strongly associated with unprofessional behavior in medical school. Students with the strongest association were those who were described as irresponsible or as having diminished ability to improve their behavior. Professionalism should have a central role in medical academics and throughout one's medical career.

Papadakis MA, Teherani A, Banach MA, et al. N Engl J Med 2005; 353(25):2673–2682.
Adapted with permission from the publisher.
For more information: http://content.nejm.org/

Medical Professionalism Project: Medical professionalism in the new millennium: a physicians' charter. Med J Aust 2002; 177(5):263–265.

Stern DT, Papadakis M. The developing physician—becoming a professional. N Engl J Med 2006; 355(17):1794–1799.

Taylor G. Clinical governance and the development of a new professionalism in medicine: educational implications. Educ Health (Abingdon) 2002; 15(1):65–70.

Thomas MR, Dyrbye LN, Huntington JL, et al. How do distress and well-being relate to medical student empathy? A multicenter study. J Gen Intern Med 2007; 22(2): 177–183.

Weaver MJ, Ow CL, Walker DJ, et al. A questionnaire for patients' evaluation of their physicians' humanistic behaviors. J Gen Intern Med 1993; 8(3):135–139.

Welie JVM. Is dentistry a profession? Part 1. Professionalism defined. J Can Dental Assoc 2004; 70(8):529–532.

Welie JVM. Is dentistry a profession? Part 2. The hallmarks of professionalism. J Can Dental Assoc 2004; 70(9):599–602.

Welie JVM. Is dentistry a profession? Part 3. Future challenges. J Can Dental Assoc 2004; 70(10):675–678.

Welling RE, Boberg JT. Professionalism: lifelong commitment for surgeons. Arch Surg 2003; 138(3):262–264.

CHAPTER 13

The 22 laws of success

> To succeed you have to believe in something with such a passion that it becomes a reality. **ANITA RODDICK**

INTRODUCTION

Success is not an accident. Success is the outcome of continuous, persistent, strategic and purposeful actions taken by you in pursuit of your goals. Your success starts with a positive state of mind, clarity of purpose and a desire to make a difference. You want your life to have an impact on your peers, your future patients, your community and everyone who works with you. You have a burning desire to achieve your potential and see your dreams come true. But there is a difference between wishing for a thing to happen and being prepared to do what is required. You are not ready until you believe deep inside you can do it.

The first step is to be open to change. Believe in your abilities and skills so you can overcome your limitations. Seeing hope and success in the middle of setbacks and failures will free you from whatever is holding you back.

Throughout history, people have achieved success by focusing on their purpose, changing their way of thinking and preparing themselves to reach their potential and enjoy life. Author and clinical psychologist, Ben Sweetland said, 'Success is a journey, not a destination'. Focus and enjoy every moment of your lifelong journey of success.

This chapter is for those who look for laws which have made others successful. Understand the 22 laws of success and apply them as you journey.

LAW 1 KNOW WHO YOU ARE

To be successful the first step is to discover yourself, to know who you are and what you really want to do with your life. Ask yourself questions like: 'What type of a person am I?', 'How do I see myself?', 'How do others see me?', 'What is my life really about?', 'Why am I studying medicine … or physiotherapy … or nursing?', 'What type of healthcare professional do I want to be?' These are empowering questions. They stimulate your thinking and help you to discover yourself.

It is important to know who you are because you want to know:
- what the driving force in your life is
- how you see yourself and your life
- what your priorities are
- what values and qualities you have
- what skills and talents you have and how you can use them

- what competencies and skills you need to learn to help you reach your potential and achieve your dreams.

LAW 2 CLARIFY YOUR PURPOSE

Successful people have meaning and purpose to their lives. But many people are not sure of their purpose. Their lives focus on the daily routine.

Your life purpose reflects what you value most in life and what you aim for. Your purpose is 'your personal mission statement'—what you would like to be chiselled on your tombstone when you end your journey of success. You should use it as the criterion by which you evaluate your life.

Your purpose is not just a statement. It is the energy that provides you with the daily fuel to work on your goals and reach your potential. It enables you to overcome obstacles you may encounter during your journey. It will strengthen your path and make you confident and clear about your priorities. Your purpose is the big picture you have of yourself—the type of person you want to be, the type of life you want to have and the type of impact you want to leave on people around you.

To be successful you need to clarify your purpose in life:

- What are you doing here?
- What do you want to achieve?
- What do you care about most?
- What are you committed to?
- What do you stand for?

LAW 3 DEFINE YOUR GOALS

We often confuse goal with purpose. A goal is not a purpose. A goal is something you want to achieve. It is something to be accomplished. A purpose is an ongoing process.

Goal setting is a powerful process for personal growth. We all need to have a clear idea of what we want to achieve, what we want to change and what we hope to see as a result of our work.

There are a number of reasons why people dislike setting goals:

- They feel that setting goals will limit their freedom.
- When they have set goals they did not work out as planned.
- They believe their priorities will change so there is no point in setting goals. Why set goals?
- You need a target to shoot at. Your goals guide your actions.
- Goal setting is essential for improvement and personal development. It is the key to reaching your potential.
- Goal setting firms your determination and sharpens your effort.
- Goals give a purpose for your actions.
- Goals foster your persistence and your ability to overcome obstacles.
- Goals help you monitor your progress and enjoy the feeling of accomplishment.
- Goals force you to make priorities, plan and use your time effectively.

Your goals should: (1) be clear, focused and specific, (2) reflect your purpose and your direction, (3) be achievable within the timeframe you have set, (4) target values that are important to you, (5) be meaningful, (6) stimulate positive actions, and (7) have a significant impact on your life once achieved.

Being clear about your goals is essential but you need to be flexible: there may be changes over time and these changes may be inevitable and beyond your control. Be flexible so you can make the appropriate changes to your plans.

LAW 4 BELIEVE IN YOUR ABILITIES

You have unlimited power. You are smart enough, creative enough and talented enough to get things to work for you. But your greatest power is in your own thinking. Your unlimited belief in yourself is your real power. Your belief about yourself and your abilities creates your expectations and desires. Your desires determine your attitude and your behaviour. Your behaviour determines how people relate to you and see you. A strong self-belief will make a good impression on those around you.

Denis Waitley once said, 'If you believe you can, you probably can. If you believe you won't, you most assuredly won't. Belief is the ignition switch that gets you off the launching pad'.

How can you use the power of thinking about yourself to create your future?

- Talk about the things you want, your dreams and your vision. Think about what will happen to your life once you achieve these dreams. Empower yourself with these thoughts every day.
- Expect the best to happen to you and it will become your own. When we feel confident that we will win, we work hard and focus on the outcomes. When we do not expect success, we are hesitant and do not put in all our effort. Positive self-expectation is a powerful key for your success.
- Program your mind for success. The power of repeated affirmation will change your thoughts, feelings, behaviour, attitude and body language. You will become what you say to yourself: positive, persistent, loving to others, capable, willing to help others, talented, skilful and willing to learn new skills.
- Take charge of your own life. Do not be shaken by setbacks or challenges. Face challenges with a winning attitude. Accept complete responsibility for yourself and your mistakes. Do not blame others or make excuses. Think about the power of this moment and how you can use it effectively. You cannot control the years that lie behind or the years that lie ahead but you can be in full control of the present moment. Get the best out of it.

LAW 5 START WITH DISCIPLINE

You cannot succeed in any walk of life without discipline. If you do not have discipline, your plans will not succeed. Having the discipline to follow through is what makes your achievements grow.

What are the components of discipline?

1 *Personal responsibility*: the ability to behave in a way that shows accountability and self-control. For example, if you value the time of others you come to meetings on time. Reflect on these questions:
   — As a student, what does personal responsibility mean to you?
   — How do you manage your time?
   — Do you come to meetings, clinical rounds, tutorials and lectures on time?
   — Do you admit it is your responsibility when things go wrong?
   — Do you miss deadlines?
   — What are the things you need to change so you can demonstrate personal responsibility?

2 *Priorities*: those things in your life that take precedence over other items. Organising time and knowing our priorities in life are key to the right results.
— What are your priorities?
— How did you reach this conclusion?
— How is knowing your priorities a component of discipline?

3 *Persistence*: the ability to hold onto your goals in the face of pressure, stress, adversity and setbacks. Persistence is refusing to give in. It is your ability to use failure and stress to come back even stronger.
— How do you perceive challenges and difficulties?
— What are your strategies when faced with difficult situations?
— What does persistence mean to you?

4 *Personal values*: what we believe in; our values determine which aspects of life we regard as important. Our values energise our actions. Examples of personal values are truth, financial gain, sophistication, wisdom, commitment, freedom, harmony, independence, family, concern for others, discipline.
— What are the values that have shaped your life?
— Which of these values will you continue to implement in your life?
— In what way can your values influence your success?

How can discipline change your life?
• The more disciplined you are, the more you multiply your rewards.
• Only through self-discipline can you achieve what you have failed to achieve in the past.
• Right discipline is in the habits of the mind; one of its products is self-respect.
• Discipline helps you make the hard decisions and stay on track despite stress, pressure and fears.
• With practice and discipline you can have confidence in your abilities and be able to avoid mistakes.
• Discipline and a sense of deep responsibility are the basis of persistence in the face of challenges and setbacks.

LAW 6 LEARN FROM FAILURE

Learning from your failures and your mistakes needs courage. Bill Gates, the master of the information age, used to publish and revise annually a memo under the title, 'The ten great mistakes of Microsoft'. His aim was not to highlight errors, but rather to stimulate everyone in the Microsoft organisation to learn from the mistakes. Learning from our mistakes and our failures is a powerful tool for achieving success and excellence.

What does failure *not* do? It does not:
• steal your skills
• stop you from trying
• prevent you from reaching your goals
• lessen your determination
• rob you of your joy.

On the other hand, failure can guide your success. Winston Churchill once said, 'Success consists of going from failure to failure without loss of enthusiasm'. Failure can empower you by:
• enhancing your experience and learning skills
• strengthening your determination to succeed

- allowing you to work more on yourself and your priorities
- teaching you wisdom.

LAW 7 PRACTISE THE ART OF COMMITMENT

Vince Lombardi Jr in his book, *What it takes to be # 1* says, 'The essence of commitment is the act of making a decision. The Latin root for "decision" is to cut away from, as an incision during surgery. When you commit to something, you are cutting away all other possibilities, all other options. When you commit to something, you are cutting away all the rationalisations, all the excuses'.

We describe people as committed when they:
- do not lose sight of their vision
- are dedicated, focused and know their path
- are able to turn their dreams, hopes and promises into a reality
- enjoy working on their projects even when there are difficulties or setbacks
- are dedicated and motivated to rise above their circumstances.

Through commitment you can:
- overcome limitations
- transform doubt into confidence and reality
- build your self-esteem and allow your vision to grow
- rise above the obstacles and challenges you face
- gain the respect you deserve from people around you.

There is no recipe for commitment and no one can help you to develop your own commitment. Commitment is something you need to develop on your own— you might struggle with yourself to maintain your commitment, so monitor your progress in your reflective journal. Learn from the feedback given to you. Persistence, willpower and self-monitoring are essential in this process.

LAW 8 LISTEN WITH YOUR HEART

Listening is a skill you can develop. The power of listening is one of the means of effective communication. If you want to be successful, work on your listening skills.

How can you improve your listening skills?
1 *Focus on the person*: although it is very important to focus on the content and the ideas being communicated, you also need to focus on the person you are communicating with. If you disagree with what was said and you have some concerns or a different view to present, you might first need to check that you understand what was said. Then:
   — acknowledge the significance of what was said and what you want to build on
   — focus on principles rather than detail
   — watch the tone of your voice and your body language: 80–90 per cent of communication is through body language
   — do not argue
   — be brief
   — ensure there is no personal bias in your opinions
   — be effective in your communication
   — never use sarcasm or inappropriate words.
2 *Avoid potential barriers*: a number of barriers can interfere with your listening.

These barriers can include:

— environmental distractors, for example, television, phone calls
— emotions: when we are too emotionally involved in listening we tend to hear what we want to hear rather than what was actually said
— pride: when we think that there is nothing significant being said, when we know better, or believe there is little to learn from others
— jumping to conclusions: when we predict or over-interpret what was communicated we may miss the point and jump to false conclusions
— interrupting: when we interrupt a lot, we do not allow the other person to pass on everything they were going to say
— lack of trust: when we lack trust, we tend not to listen carefully and become sarcastic or underestimate the significance of what was said.

3 *Focus on understanding.*

4 *Turn listening into an active and challenging mental task.*

LAW 9 WORK ON YOUR ATTITUDE

Who you are is not determined by the degrees you have, where you live, how you look or who your friends are. Your attitude determines who you are. Your attitude is your habit of thoughts; how you perceive things, what you think about yourself and others, how you deal with challenging situations, how you see opportunities. Therefore, if you want to change your attitude, you must change the way you think.

What are the effects of your attitude on your life?

• Your attitude determines how you see challenges and perceive difficult situations. A positive attitude makes you focus on solutions and success, rather than on setbacks or stress.

• Your attitude determines how you see your abilities and skills. A positive attitude gives you confidence and the willingness to achieve and succeed.

• Your attitude affects how you see others. People with a negative attitude do not trust people working with them and think of competition rather than collaboration. People with a positive attitude foster the self-esteem of people working with them, enjoy working with others and invest in their relationships with others.

• Your attitude determines how you see success and your potential for success. People with a negative attitude doubt their ability to succeed, expect failure, blame circumstances and make excuses. People with a positive attitude expect success. They focus and use self-motivation to accomplish their goals.

How can you create a positive attitude?

• You can change your attitude if you change the way you think. Focus on statements such as, 'I want to think in a positive way even when circumstances are not good', 'I want to be constructive', 'I want to change the way I think about …', 'I want to make a positive impact'. Such statements can stimulate your thinking and engage you as you change and shape the way you think.

• Work on your thoughts, your speech patterns and behaviour.

• Visualise the impact of positive attitudes on yourself and the people around you. Reflect on how these changes can affect your life and the opportunities that may become available to you as a result.

• Reinforce new attitudes by practising them each day. Monitor your progress and what you have learnt.

LAW 10 OFFER YOUR VERY BEST

When you give your very best to others, you invest in them, showing them how much you care. You strengthen your relationships with others, you make a positive impact on them and you feel fulfilled. As you practise this attitude you will build your own character; you will become less selfish.

Why do you want to offer your very best to others?
- by offering your very best to others, you are more able to engage with them
- by putting other people first and treating them with respect, you build trust and cultivate strong relationships with them
- by offering your very best, you will enjoy a return in due time. It will come in unexpected ways and you will be moved by the response.

LAW 11 REPLACE BAD HABITS WITH GOOD ONES

A bad habit is an acquired pattern of behaviour you cannot control. Any habit can become a bad habit, starting out as an attractive thing to do, then slowly beginning to sour. Once a bad habit takes hold, it can be destructive. Bad habits take many forms:
- lying to save your own skin or protect others
- showing carelessness towards others
- losing your temper
- being chronically late
- blaming others for your problems
- neglecting your health
- gambling, smoking, taking drugs
- negative thinking
- wasting your time
- procrastination and lack of organisation.

How do bad habits kill your dreams? They:
- prevent you from reaching your personal potential. They drain your money, time, energy and motivation. They hold you back from reaching your goals
- may interfere with your credibility and damage your self-image
- can be obstacles to your pursuit of happiness.

The process you use to break a bad habit is the same no matter what type of habit you are dealing with. The bottom line is you need to change the way you think before undertaking any action.
- Start with one habit that you really want to change. Think about the consequences of your bad habit; how this habit can damage your dream.
- Identify the good habit you want to acquire instead.
- Think about successful people you know who possess this good habit. Reflect on the impact this habit has on their lives.
- Focus on the ingredients of the good habit you desire to have for your success. Learn more about this habit. Read biographies of successful people and examine this habit more closely.
- Start working on the good habit now. Do it now. Put it into practice.
- Remember that changing to a successful habit will not happen overnight: you need to work hard on yourself to achieve your goal. You might need somebody to support you even though the main reason for success will be how hard you work on yourself.

LAW 12 RECOGNISE THE POWER OF PREPARATION

One of the keys for building your confidence is preparation. Why is preparation essential for your success?

1 Great success is often determined by the depth of knowledge, skills, qualities and attitudes you have. Preparation gives you the opportunity to master the detail, practise skills, develop good habits and demonstrate a positive attitude. Continuous preparation is the way for great success.

2 Preparation gives you the opportunity to prepare your thoughts, search for information, ask new questions and search for answers, see the big picture as well as the fine details and develop the competencies needed for future challenges.

3 Without preparation and giving yourself enough time to assess a situation, you will not be able to deliver the right actions. This could lead to failure. Good preparation will provide you with the opportunity to carefully study every possibility, weigh the evidence for each option and make the right decision before taking action.

4 Preparation provides you with the opportunity to refine your decisions and identify changes you need to make to your plan.

5 Preparation allows you to learn new techniques, accept new ideas, seek the input and opinions of others and become more flexible in your approach.

LAW 13 BE READY FOR CHANGE

Change is a constant and affects us in all facets of our lives: as individuals, in families, communities and organisations, and at local, national and global levels.

Here are some of the changes you might face as a student in a problem-based learning (PBL) course:

- Learning may require new learning strategies (for example, small-group discussion, self-directed learning, and collaborative learning).
- Assessment tools used in the course may be new to you (for example, MCQs, EMQs, PBL-style questions, OSCE).
- The course may require learning and using hundreds of medical and scientific terminology words.
- The course may require competency in the English language, which could be a challenge if you are from a non-English-speaking background.
- The course may require you to master new skills and competencies.
- The culture embedded in the course may be different to what you are used to.

Change is a natural process that we have to accept. We also have to accept the feelings that accompany it. Even more importantly, we have to adapt ourselves to the consequences of the change. Here are some responses to change:

1 *Be in control*:
  — If the situation is frustrating, control your anger.
  — Give yourself a break, take time off to relax.
  — If possible, avoid other sources of stress.
  — Think of activities you can do to help renew your energy, for example, drawing, sports, spiritual activities.
  — Prepare yourself on a daily basis for other challenges.

2 *Reflect*: reflect upon what you have learnt from the situation. Think about how you can use the situation to reach your goals and turn it into a successful moment.

3 *Reorganise your schedule*: the stress caused by the change may necessitate rescheduling to take time to relax. Perhaps one of your friends will keep you updated on lectures and tutorials you have missed.

4 *Ask for help*: the change may bring with it negative thinking, blame, depression, a sense of vulnerability and grief. You might feel powerless and need help. Friends and family members can be a great help. You might also share your fears and worries with your mentor or tutor.

5 *Stay focused on the big picture and your purpose*: all successful people are challenged with changes, problems and setbacks—more than you might imagine. Stay focused on what you planned.

LAW 14 EXTEND YOUR LIMITS

During your journey of success, numerous opportunities to extend your skills will become available. These opportunities may give you a chance to go where you have never gone before and grow through the experience.

Extending your limits can take various forms, for example:

- undertaking a research project during your undergraduate years in a university overseas
- undertaking a combined degree such as medicine and law or physiotherapy and arts
- travelling to another country to do part of your internship
- volunteering to work in an African country during an end-of-year holiday.

The British novelist, Arnold Bennett wrote, 'The real tragedy is the tragedy of the man who never in his life braces himself for his one supreme effort—he never stretches to his full capacity, never stands up to his full stature'. You need to face your fears and take risks. You also need commitment, to believe in yourself, think big, and liberate yourself from whatever holds you back.

Pursuing your dreams will never happen unless you decide to leave your comfort zone and to move into new unsecured territory where you have less control. The aim is to expand your comfort zone by making the unknown known. This will help you develop new skills and discover the hidden talents you have. If you do not leave your comfort zone you may miss out on the best opportunities to deepen your experiences and extend your success.

LAW 15 PUT OFF PROCRASTINATION

Procrastination is not just the thief of time, it is one of the biggest obstacles to decision making. People put things off to avoid experiencing failure. They believe they are better off not trying.

How can you put off procrastination?

- *Take one step at a time*: large projects cannot be completed in a short time. If you procrastinate you will never work on them. Start now. If you do a small part each day, you will overcome your procrastination.
- *Be in control*: the real battle of procrastination is in the mind and directly related to negative thoughts. The procrastinator develops a sense of helplessness and victimisation. This can hold them back from doing anything. If you face a similar situation, you need to free yourself from these thoughts and focus on the outcomes and rewards you will receive.

- *Start now*: there is no better time than now. Sit down and start the process. You might need to force yourself to get started. Plan what you will do next and how you will manage the whole task.
- *Do not rely on tomorrow*: procrastinators think that they will be able to manage their work tomorrow. They say to themselves, 'Tomorrow there will be more time to start working on these tasks. Today I am very busy and not in a good mood to do such things'. They never find a suitable day to start working on their projects. The only solution to this is to begin working now.
- *Focus on rewards*: procrastinators think about the pain and demands associated with doing a task. They do not think about the rewards of taking action, the outcomes of their work and the impact on their lives or the pleasure they might experience while working on their task. How many times have we felt that a task will be difficult, only to discover that it was not as painful as expected?
- *Ask for help*: if you cannot manage on your own, you might need a coach or a support person who can work with you to rid you of your procrastination and assist you in organising your work.

LAW 16 REALISE THE POWER OF MAKING GOOD DECISIONS

One of the keys for success is the ability to make good decisions. Are you a good decision maker?

Good decisions:
- provide you with new opportunities
- make you feel good about yourself
- enhance your potential
- allow you to achieve your goals
- expand your skills and talents
- reduce your frustration and put you back on the road to success
- provide an opportunity to move to the next stage of your journey of success
- motivate you to continue working and successfully complete a task
- allow you to extend your limits
- make a positive impact on your life
- energise you to focus on specific objectives
- force you to use your time effectively.

Decision making is a skill that can be learnt. Good decisions are usually made by carefully considering all options and periodically assessing the decision and its effects.

The following seven steps can help you make good decisions:

1 *Challenge*: ask yourself if this is really your decision or if it is for someone else to decide. If it is yours, then

2 *Brainstorm*: write down as many options as you can think of.

3 *Research*: find more information about each option.

4 *Evaluate*: list the outcomes of each option. Take the emotion out of the decision process. You do not want to base your decision on your feelings. If you rush to make your evaluation you may choose a solution that does not fit with your values.

5 *Rank*: assess each item in your list and put them into three groups: 1—most likely, 2—less likely and 3—to be crossed off.

6 *Focus*: carefully assess all the options that fit with the situation.

7 *Decide*: consolidate the objectives that support your final decision.

LAW 17 MONITOR YOUR PROGRESS

The skills and competencies we have that are rated as 'good' should become even better as we progress. If they don't, we will be moving backwards rather than forwards on our journey. What causes people to move backwards rather than forwards?

*   When things go well, people become overconfident. They focus on their past accomplishments. They slow down and become less able to see what they need to do to move forward.
*   When things go well, people become overly confident that they have done a good job. They lose insight about the need to introduce changes, learn new techniques and master skills.
*   Some people become less flexible and fail to change their strategies. For example, a graduate-entry student studying medicine in a PBL curriculum needs to be flexible and willing to change their learning style to suit the needs of the curriculum.
*   People fail to grow when they do not move from their comfort zone. They fail to take new directions; instead they follow a predetermined path based on what they have already done.

LAW 18 REALISE THE POWER OF SKILFUL THINKING

Skilful thinking is vital for your success. If you ask successful people the one thing that changed their life, many would say 'my life changed when I realised I needed to change the way I think'. To achieve progress, successful people embrace skilful thinking as an essential component of their daily lifestyle.

With the rapid accumulation of new knowledge, you might find it challenging to keep up-to-date. Lifelong learning has become a priority in most professions. As the singer Eartha Kitt said, 'I am learning all the time. The tombstone will be my diploma'. However, what is important is not the quantity of knowledge you know, it is your ability to think well. What type of resources do you need to read? How can these resources be of help? How can you use this new information? What else do you need to know?

Learning how to think well to achieve your goals and reach your potential is vital. Take a look at just a few reasons why you need skilful thinking:

1 *Skilful thinking is empowering*: successful people empower themselves through their thinking. Their thoughts and actions guide them to produce good results. When we focus our minds on skilful thinking:
    — our attitudes mirror our minds and the way we think
    — we feel more confident and energetic
    — our minds create more good and creative thoughts
    — we build up people around us
    — we find solutions in the midst of problems and setbacks.

2 *Skilful thinking keeps you focused on your goals*: the more you use your mind to reflect on your goals and plans, the more you will create new and useful thoughts for tomorrow's challenges.

3 *Skilful thinking increases your compassion*: it can change the way you see the world, your priorities and your compassion towards humanity.

4 *Skilful thinking enhances your problem-solving skills*: to solve problems you need critical thinking, analytical skills, enquiry planning and lateral thinking. You also need to think about new solutions and creative ideas that can provide you with optimal solutions. Yesterday's solutions may not be ideal; only through creative thinking can you generate new hypotheses and seek innovative ideas that enable you to challenge routine solutions developed in the past by a particular experience.

5 *Skilful thinking increases your opportunities*: opportunities will not come if you wait for them. Successful people do not wait for things to happen; they create their own opportunities.

LAW 19 REALISE THE POWER OF TODAY

Many people believe that success means hard work; working day and night to produce as much as they can. Although hard work is vital, many people who work hard never realise success. Some work so hard they damage important relationships and their health, lose interest and burn out or fail to reach their potential.

Others let negative experiences shape them for their entire lives. If you are one of those people I say, 'Yesterday is not in your hands any more. It ended at midnight'. You cannot do anything to change yesterday or get back a second from yesterday. If there is nothing constructive that you have learnt from yesterday, do not take any burden from the past to disturb today.

The same is true for tomorrow. Do not overestimate or underestimate what tomorrow can bring you. You do not know whether tomorrow will be better or worse for you. Worrying about tomorrow will not help you.

Therefore the only time left for you is today. Today is your great investment. Focus on today and get the best out of each minute you have.
- Stay focused and productive.
- Learn new skills and seek to improve your competencies.
- Empower others and motivate people around you.
- Build relationships and serve others.
- Work on your goals, move forward and learn new good habits.

 Effective use of today will help you to:
- prepare for tomorrow
- invest in important competencies such as time management and managing priorities
- enjoy what you are doing and experience fulfilment.

LAW 20 DEAL WITH THE REAL SOURCE OF OBSTACLES

When people face obstacles and setbacks, they often blame circumstances, authority figures or the lack of resources. There is no value in blaming. This attitude drains energy and will never get you moving towards your goals.

We all know how powerful the mind is in helping us achieve our goals and reach our potential. But sometimes the mind can become the source of our trouble and the biggest barrier to good performance, resulting in anxiety, nagging thoughts, lack of focus, doubts, fears and poor performance. Remember that the mind is the:
- heart of the emotions and feelings
- treasure chest of the memories
- energy store of the enthusiasm, determination and resilience
- creative theatre for the thoughts, imaginations and dreams

- executive room for making decisions and generating strategies
- directory for establishing connections with others.

The great challenge is how we perceive obstacles and how we deal with our mental barriers. Our fears, anxiety, hesitation, loss of self-control and inability to make the right decision create damage and keep us in a state of continuous loss. When we take personal responsibility and put in the effort wisely, we will reap the benefits of self-fulfilment and self-confidence. We will also overcome obstacles.

LAW 21 DEVELOP PERSISTENCE SKILLS

Your ability to respond effectively to setbacks, difficulties, unexpected crises, and temporary failure will make a significant difference to your life. There is no success without temporary failure. Unexpected health problems, family crises, difficulties in relationships and financial problems are just some of the unavoidable problems that can happen to all of us.

Our ability to respond effectively to such situations and how we turn them into opportunities for success will have a major impact on our lives and our ability to succeed. With persistence you will win. Persistence is the energy that empowers you to visualise your success even when the odds are against you.

When there is a lack of persistence, people:
- procrastinate and lose opportunities
- blame others and circumstances for their failure
- lose their desire to work and achieve
- lose direction
- become hesitant, wishing rather than doing
- lose their vision and become undecided.

How to develop persistence:
1 *Clarify your purpose*: review your personal mission statement and clarify your purpose. Believe in what you are doing.
2 *Design an action plan* that allows you to work on your goals and turn your dreams into a reality.
3 *Use feedback* given to you by your peers, tutors, supervisors, or coaches to identify areas of weakness that you need to work on.
4 *Eliminate negative thoughts*: focus on constructive and positive thoughts. Positive thoughts lead to positive feelings. Enjoy what you are doing. Visualise your success.
5 *Seek support and encouragement*: if you feel that you cannot manage on your own, seek help.
6 *Monitor your progress*: review the progress you have made, identify the obstacles and challenges you face and how you can manage them.

LAW 22 HAPPINESS IS A CHOICE

People do not agree on what makes happiness. When we search for what great thinkers said about happiness, we find many opinions: Aristotle linked happiness with the meaning and purpose of life, Thomas Jefferson saw it in human relationships, Victor Hugo saw that the greatest happiness is to be convinced you are loved and Abraham Lincoln linked happiness to how we make up our minds.

Whatever the definition is, happiness is very significant to everyone. There is a strong body of research evidence that variations in happiness have an impact on a range of our day-to-day activities, creativity, engagement in activities, satisfaction levels, absenteeism (from school, university, workplace), and achievements. Therefore, the last law is about enjoying life now and choosing to be happy today. You don't need to wait for optimal circumstances to feel happy. You do not need to link happiness with the achievement of your goals, reaching the body size you want or fixing a broken relationship. Think about happiness as a choice. You choose to feel happy as you start your day. You may be going through tough times, difficulties or challenges and you may have compelling reasons not to be happy. But being unhappy will not solve your problem or change the situation. You can instead choose to feel happy, enjoy your life and empower yourself.

Here are some ways to stay happy:

- Make the most of every moment.
- Do not be disturbed by little things and daily minor troubles. Do not lose your peace.
- See the best in every situation and every person.
- Accept people as they are.
- Make others feel happy—people like to feel they are unique.
- Enjoy what you are doing.
- Do not worry about things you cannot change.
- Keep a positive attitude.
- Smile often.
- Build trust and help others grow.

CONCLUSIONS

By putting these laws of success into practice, you provide yourself with every opportunity to reach your maximum potential. You are preparing yourself to be the person that everyone would like to work with and you will have a clear vision of your purpose and what you need to do to fulfil your dreams.

FURTHER READING
BOOKS

Blanchard K, Peal NV. The power of ethical management: you don't have to cheat to win. London: Heinemann Kingswood; 1988.

Burley-Allen M. Listening: The forgotten skill: a self-teaching guide. New York: John Wiley & Sons Ltd; 1995.

Canfield J. How to get from where you are to where you want to be: the 25 principles of success. Sydney: HarperCollins; 2005.

Carson B, Murphey C. Think big: unleashing your potential for excellence. Grand Rapids, Michigan: Zondervan Publishing House; 1992.

Center for Association Leadership. 7 measures of success: what remarkable associations do that others don't. Washington, DC: ASAE & Center for Association Leadership; 2006.

Chopra D. The seven spiritual laws of success. New York: New World Library; 1995.

Covey SR. The 7 habits of highly effective people. New York: Fireside; 1990.

Covey SR. The 8th habit: from effectiveness to greatness. New York: Free Press; 2004.

De Bono E. The happiness purpose. Middlesex: Penguin Books; 1977.

Gates B. Business @ the speed of thoughts: using a digital nervous system. Ringwood, Vic: Viking; 1999.

Hill N. Law of success: the 21st-century edition: revised and updated. New York: Penguin; 2004.

Hill N. Napoleon Hill's keys to success: the 17 principles of personal achievement. New York: Penguin; 1994.

Hill N, Stone WC. Success through a positive mental attitude. New York: Pocket Books; 1991.

Kratz DM, Kratz AR. Effective listening skills. Boston: McGraw-Hill; 1995.

Lombardi V, Jr. What it takes to be # 1: Vince Lombardi on leadership. New York: McGraw-Hill; 2001.

Maxwell JC. Success one day at a time journal. Nashville: Thomas Nelson; 2000.

Maxwell JC. Winning with people. Tennessee: Nelson; 2004.

Maxwell JC. The 360 degree leader. Tennessee: Nelson; 2005.

Meyer PJ. 24 keys that bring complete success. Florida: Bridge-Logos; 2006.

Newberry T. Success is not an accident: change your choice, change your life. Oregon: Looking Glass Books; 1999.

Osteen J. Your best life now: 7 steps to living at your full potential. New York: Warner; 2004.

Porras J, Emery S, Thompson M. Success built to last: creating a life that matters. Upper Saddle River, NJ: Wharton School Publishing; 2007.

Schwartz DJ. The magic of thinking big: Acquiring the secrets of success, achieve everything you have always wanted. New York: Simon & Schuster; 1990.

Simmons JG. Doctors and discoveries: lives that created today's medicine. New York: Houghton Mifflin; 2002.

Starzel TE. The puzzle people: memories of a transplant surgeon. An autobiography of Dr Thomas Starzel. Pittsburgh: The University of Pittsburgh Press; 1992.

Templar R. The rules of work: a definitive code for personal success. London: Pearson Education; 2003.

Thomas VT. Partners of the heart: Vivien Thomas and his work with Alfred Blalock. An autobiography of Vivien T. Thomas. Philadelphia: University of Pennsylvania Press; 1998.

Tracy B. Maximum achievement. New York: Simon & Schuster; 1993.

Tracy B. Goals! San Francisco: Berrett-Koehler Publishers; 2003.

Tracy B. Change your thinking; change your life. Upper Saddle River, NJ: John Wiley & Sons Ltd; 2005.

Waitley D. Being the best. New York: Pocket Books; 1987.

Warren R. The purpose driven life. Grand Rapids, Michigan: Zondervan Publishing House; 2002.

Williams P, Williams R, Mink M. How to be like women of influence: life lessons from 20 of the greatest. Florida: Health Communications; 2003.

Zaslove MO. The successful physician: a productivity handbook for practitioners. Boston: Jones and Bartlett Publishers: 2003.

Ziglar Z. Over the top. Revised & updated. Nashville: Thomas Nelson; 1997.

ARTICLES AND RESEARCH PAPERS

Gunderman RB. Why do some people succeed where others fail? Implications for education. Radiology 2003; 226(1):29–31.

King L, Napa C. What makes a life good? J Pers Soc Psychol 1998; 75(1):156–165.

Kisfalvi V. The threat of failure, the perils of success and CEO character: sources of strategic persistence. Organ Stud 2000; 21(3):611–639.

Lee FK, Sheldon KM, Turban DB. Personality and the goal-striving process: The influence of achievement goal patterns, goal level, and mental focus on performance and enjoyment. J Appl Psychol 2003; 88(2):256–265.

Appendix A

RECOMMENDED ONLINE RESOURCES

Clinical education
eMedicine: http://www.emedicine.com
Harrison's Online: http://www.harrisonsonline.com
Mayo Clinic: http://www.mayoclinic.com/
Med BioWorld: http://www.medbioworld.com/index.html
Medem: http://www.medem.com/search/default.cfm
Medical Matrix: http://www.medmatrix.org/reg/login.asp
MedicineNet: http://www.medicinenet.com/script/main/hp.asp
MedicineOnline: http://www.medicineonline.com
Medscape: http://www.medscape.com/cardiology
MedWeb: http://170.140.250.52/MedWeb/ http
Merck*Medicus*: http://www.merckmedicus.com/pp/us/hcp/hcp_home.jsp
National Cancer Institute (US): http://www.cancer.gov/
Virology Journal: http://www.tulane.edu/~dmsander/garryfavweb.html

Drug information
Drug information (PDR Health): http://www.pdrhealth.com/drug_info/index.
    html
Drug resource centre (Aetna IntliHealth): http://www.intelihealth.com/IH/
    ihtIH/WSIHW000/8124/8124.html?k=menuxx408x8124

Biomedical science
Gross anatomy (University of Arkansas for Medical Sciences): http://anatomy.
    uams.edu/anatomyhtml/gross_atlas.html
Gross anatomy, atlas images (University of Michigan Medical School): http://
    anatomy.med.umich.edu/atlas/atlas_index.html
Interactive anatomy atlas (University of Washington): http://www9.biostr.
    washington.edu/da.html
Atlas of echocardiogram—heart anatomy (Yale University): http://www.med.yale.
    edu/intmed/cardio/echo_atlas/references/heart_anatomy.html
Neuroanatomy tutorials (Florida State University College of Medicine): http://
    medlib.med.utah.edu/WebPath/HISTHTML/NEURANAT/NEURANCA.
    html
Neuroanatomy atlas (State University of New York): http://ect.downstate.edu/
    courseware/neuro_atlas/
Neuroanatomy structures: http://www.neuropat.dote.hu/anastru/anastru.htm
Neuroanatomy atlas (National Academy of Neuropsychology): http://schatz.sju.
    edu/neuro/NeuroFound/
Martindales's anatomy & histology center: http://www.martindalecenter.com/
    MedicalAnatomy_3_SAD.html
The Urbana Atlas of Pathology (University of Illinois): http://www.med.uiuc.edu/
    pathatlasf/

Pathology Atlas of Gross and Microscopic Images (Columbia University Health Sciences):http://cait.cpmc.columbia.edu:88/dept/curric-pathology/ pathology/pathology/pathoatlas/index.html

Pathweb, University of Connecticut's virtual pathology museum: http://pathweb. uchc.edu/

McGill University histopathology website: http://sprojects.mmi.mcgill.ca/ histopathology/histopathologyMS.htm

Pathology Education Resources Laboratory, Indiana University: http://erl. pathology.iupui.edu/INDEX.HTM

Clinical cases and pathology images

The University of New South Wales Museum of Human Disease: http://web.med. unsw.edu.au/pathmus/

Leicester University The Virtual Autopsy: http://www.le.ac.uk/pathology/teach/ va/titlpag1.html

University of Pittsburgh Department of Pathology case studies: http://path.upmc. edu/cases.html

Gastrointestinal endoscopy

Atlas of Gastrointestinal Endoscopy (Atlanta South Gastroenterology): http:// www.endoatlas.com/

Atlas of Gastroenterological Endoscopy (A Freytag, T Deist): http://www. endoskopischer-atlas.de/indexe.htm

Video Atlas Gastrointestinal Endoscopy with cases (J Murra-Saca): http://www. murrasaca.com/Videoatlas.htm

Clinical Cases and Endoscopy Images (G Hawken): http://www.endoscopyatlas. com/

Medical dictionaries

Medical Abbreviations Dictionary (mediLexicon): http://www.medilexicon.com/ medicalabbreviations.php

Online Medical Dictionary (University of Newcastle upon Tyne): http:// cancerweb.ncl.ac.uk/omd/index.html

MedTerms Medical Dictionary (MedicineNet): http://www.medterms.com/ script/main/hp.asp

Merriam-Webster Medical Dictionary (Medline Plus): http://medlineplus.nlm. nih.gov/medlineplus/mplusdictionary.html

Medline Plus Medical Encyclopaedia: http://www.nlm.nih.gov/medlineplus/ encyclopedia.html

General

Centers for Disease Control and Prevention: http://www.cdc.gov/

NOAH (consumer health information of high quality): http://www.noah-health. org/

The United States National Library of Medicine: http://www.nlm.nih.gov/

BioEthicsWeb (Intute: Health & Life Sciences): http://www.intute.ac.uk/ healthandlifesciences/bioethicsweb/

AARP internet resources on ageing: http://www.aarp.org

The Cochrane Collaboration (Reviews and library): http://www.cochrane.org/
reviews/clibintro.htm
MDchoice.com (Medical information library for all students of medicine): www.
medicalstudent.com
Merck and the Merck Manuals: http://www.merck.com/pubs/
MedicalMnemonics: http://www.medicalmnemonics.com/
FreeBooks4Doctors: http://freebooks4doctors.com/index.htm
Hardin Library (Medical/health sciences libraries on the web): www.lib.uiowa.
edu/hardin/
Medical statistics: http://bmj.bmjjournals.com/statsbk/
World Health Report (World Health Organization): http://www.who.int/whr/
en/

Health organisations
Directory of Health Organisations: http://dirline.nlm.nih.gov/
Worldwide hospitals directory: http://www.medilexicon.com/hospitalsdirectory.
php
Medical associations and societies: http://www.medilexicon.com/
medicalassociations.php

Appendix B

RECOMMENDED TEXTBOOKS AND JOURNALS

Textbooks

Abbas AK, Lichtman AH. Cellular and molecular immunology. 5th edn. New York: Saunders; 2003.

Ackermann U. PDQ Physiology. Hamilton: BC Decker Inc; 2002.

Agur AMR, Lee MJ. Grant's atlas of anatomy. 10th edn. Philadelphia: Lippincott Williams & Wilkins; 2000.

Azer SA. Core clinical cases in basic biomedical science. London: Hodder Arnold; 2006

Basmajian JV, Slonecker CE. Grant's method of anatomy. 11th edn. Baltimore: Williams & Wilkins; 1989.

Bennett PN, Brown MJ. Clinical pharmacology. 9th edn. Edinburgh: Churchill Livingstone; 2003.

Bhagavan NV. Medical biochemistry. 4th edn. San Diego: Harcourt/Academic Press; 2002.

Boron WF, Boulpaep EL. Medical physiology. Updated edn. Philadelphia: Saunders; 2005.

Chandrasoma P, Taylor CR. Concise pathology. 3rd edn. Stamford: Appleton & Lange; 1998.

Craig CR, Stitzel RE. Modern pharmacology with clinical applications. 6th edn. Philadelphia: Lippincott Williams & Wilkins; 2004.

Damjanov I, Linder J. Anderson's pathology. 10th edn. St Louis: Mosby; 1996.

Davis A, Blakeley AGH, Kidd C. Human physiology. Edinburgh: Churchill Livingstone; 2001.

Dornan T, O'Neill P. Core clinical skills for OSCE in medicine. 2nd edn. Edinburgh: Churchill Livingstone; 2006.

Drake RL, Vogl W, Mitchell AWM. Gray's anatomy for students. Philadelphia: Elsevier Churchill Livingstone; 2005.

Gartner LP, Hiatt JL. Color textbook of histology. 3rd edn. New York: Saunders; 2007.

Goldman L, Ausiello D. Cecil textbook of medicine. 22nd edn. New York: Saunders; 2004.

Greenspan FS, Gardner DG. Basic and clinical endocrinology. 7th edn. New York: Lange Medical Books/McGraw-Hill; 2004.

Guyton AC, Hall JE. Textbook of medical physiology. 11th edn. Philadelphia: Saunders; 2000.

Hardmann JG, Limbird LE. Goodman & Gilman's the pharmacological basis of therapeutics. 11th edn. New York: McGraw-Hill; 2005.

Johnson LR. Essential medical physiology. 3rd edn. Philadelphia: Elsevier; 2003.

Jorde LB, Carey JC, Bamshad MJ, et al. Medical genetics. 3rd edn. St Louis: Mosby; 2006.

Junqueira LC, Carneiro J. Basic histology: text and atlas. 10th edn. New York: Lange Medical Books/McGraw-Hill; 2004.

Kandel ER, Schwartz JH, Jessel TM. Principles of neural science. 4th edn. New York: McGraw-Hill; 2000.

Katzung BG. Basic and clinical pharmacology. 9th edn. New York: McGraw-Hill; 2004.

Kierszenbaum AL. Histology and cell biology. 2nd edn. St Louis: Mosby; 2007.

Kumar P, Clark M. Clinical medicine. 6th edn. Edinburgh: Saunders; 2005.

Kushner TK and Thomasma DC (eds). Ward ethics. Cambridge: Cambridge University Press; 2001.

Larsen P, Kronenburg H, Melmed S, et al. Williams textbook of endocrinology. 10th edn. Philadelphia: WB Saunders; 2003.

Lilly LS. Pathophysiology of heart disease. A collaborative project of medical students and faculty. 3rd edn. Philadelphia: Lippincott Williams & Wilkins; 2003.

Lloyd M, Bor R. Communication skills for medicine. 2nd edn. Edinburgh: Churchill Livingstone; 2004.

Mandell GL, Bennett JE, Dolin R. Principles and practice of infectious diseases. 6th edn. New York: Churchill Livingstone; 2005.

McPhee SJ, Lingappa VR, Ganong WF. Pathophysiology of disease. An introduction to clinical medicine. 6th edn. New York: Lange Medical Books/McGraw-Hill; 2005.

Mims C, Dockrell HM, Goering RV, et al. Medical microbiology. 3rd edn. St Louis: Mosby; 2005.

Moore KL, Dalley AF. Clinically oriented anatomy. 5th edn. Philadelphia: Lippincott Williams & Wilkins; 2005.

Murray RK, Granner DK, Mayer PA, et al. Harper's illustrated biochemistry. 26th edn. New York: McGraw-Hill; 2003.

Nolte J. The human brain. An introduction to its functional anatomy. 5th edn. St Louis: Mosby; 2002.

Page C, Hoffman B, Curtis M, et al. Integrated pharmacology. 3rd edn. Edinburgh: Mosby; 2006.

Pollard TD, Earnshaw WC, Lippincott-Schwartz J. Cell biology. 2nd edn. New York: Saunders; 2007.

Rubin R, Strayer DS. Rubin's pathology. 5th edn. Philadelphia: Lippincott Williams & Wilkins; 2007.

Rudolph AM, Kamei RK, Overby KJ. Rudolph's fundamentals of pediatrics. 3rd edn. New York: McGraw-Hill; 2002.

Souhami RL, Moxham J. Textbook of medicine. 4th edn. Edinburgh: Churchill Livingstone; 2003.

Symonds I, Baker P, Kean L. Problem oriented obstetrics & gynaecology. London: Hodder Arnold; 2002.

Underwood JCE. General and systematic pathology. 4th edn. Edinburgh: Churchill Livingstone; 2004.

Williamson RCN, Waxman BP. Scott: an aid to clinical surgery. 6th edn. Edinburgh: Churchill Livingstone; 1998.

Young B, Lowe J, Stevens A, et al. Wheater's functional histology. 5th edn. New York: Churchill Livingstone; 2006.

Young PA, Young PH. Basic clinical neuroanatomy. Philadelphia: Lippincott Williams & Wilkins; 1996.

Clinical and scientific medical journals

(These journals are available in your medical library)

American Family Physician: http://www.aafp.org/online/en/home.html

Annals of Internal Medicine: http://www.annals.org/

Archives of Family Medicine: http://archfami.ama-assn.org/

Archives of Internal Medicine: http://archinte.ama-assn.org/

Australian Family Physician: http://www.racgp.org.au/afp

British Journal of General Practice: http://www.rcgp.org.uk/journal_/bjgp.aspx

BMJ (British Medical Journal): http://bmj.bmjjournals.com/

Canadian Family Physician: http://www.cfpc.ca/cfp/2006/Sep/cover.asp?

Canadian Medical Association Journal: http://www.cmaj.ca/

Evidence-Based Medicine (American College of Physicians): http://ebm.
   bmjjournals.com/

Journal of the American Medical Association (JAMA): http://jama.ama-assn.org/

Journal of Family Medicine On-Line: http://www.ccspublishing.com/j_fammed.
   htm

Journal of Obstetrics and Gynecology: http://www.ccspublishing.com/j_obg.htm

Medical Journal of Australia: http://www.mja.com.au/

New Zealand Family Physician: http://www.rnzcgp.org.nz/

The Lancet: http://www.thelancet.com/

The New England Journal of Medicine: http://content.nejm.org/

Appendix C

EXAMPLES OF WELL-PREPARED LEARNING ISSUES
(see Ch 7, p. 122)

How are lipids transported in the body?

Cholesterol and triacylglycerols (TG) are transported in the bloodstream and other body fluids in the form of lipoprotein particles. Because lipids are hydrophobic (not soluble in blood and water), they are surrounded by a shell of more polar lipids and protein, making them more hydrophilic (soluble in water). These protein components are called apoproteins. The apoproteins have two main functions:

1 solubilise hydrophobic lipids
2 contain cell-targeting signals.

The main lipoproteins

> Chylomicrons
> Very low density lipoproteins (VLDL)
> Intermediate density lipoproteins (IDL)
> Low density lipoprotein (LDL)
> High density lipoproteins (HDL)

Apolipoproteins

Apolipoproteins are synthesised and secreted by the liver (e.g. B-100) and the intestine (e.g. B-48). The functions of apolipoproteins are:

1 activation of enzyme lipoprotein lipase (e.g. C-II)
2 inhibition of enzyme lipoprotein lipase (e.g. C-III)
3 binding a lipoprotein to a receptor (e.g. Apo-E present in IDL helps in binding IDL to LDL receptors)
4 activation of lecithin–cholesterol acyltransferase (LCAT) (e.g. Apo A-I).

Types of apolipoproteins

> A: A-I (activates LCAT), present in HDL and chylomicrons
> A-II present in HDL and chylomicrons
> B: B-100 (formed in the liver), present in VLDL, IDL and LDL
> B-48 (formed in the intestine), present in chylomicrons and remnant chylomicrons
> C: C-II (activates lipoprotein lipase), present in chylomicrons, VLDL, IDL and HDL
> C-III (inhibits lipoprotein lipase), present in chylomicrons, VLDL, IDL and HDL
> E: (legend for binding IDL and remnant chylomicrons to LDL receptors), present in chylomicrons, VLDL, IDL and HDL

Important conclusions

1 The only apolipoprotein for LDL is B-100 (it has no other apolipoproteins). What is the significance of this information?
2 C-II, C-III and E are all present in chylomicrons, VLDL, IDL and HDL.
3 A-I and A-II are present in HDL and chylomicrons. What is the significance of this information?
4 B-100 is present on VLDL, IDL and LDL.

TABLE 1 Lipoproteins and their metabolism

Property	Chylomicrons (CM)	Very low density lipoproteins (VLDL)	Intermediate density lipoproteins (IDL)	Low density lipoproteins (LDL)	High density lipoproteins (HDL)
Site of synthesis	Intestine	Liver and intestine	Mainly blood	In blood and liver from IDL and VLDL	Liver and intestine
Functions	Transport of dietary fat from intestine to the liver and adipose tissue. The triglyceride element is hydrolysed by lipoprotein lipase and the cholesterol-rich part is taken by the liver	Transport of endogenous triglycerides from the liver. Triglycerides are degraded by lipoprotein lipase resulting in the production of IDL	50% of the formed IDL are taken by the liver from the circulation 2–6 h after their formation. The remaining 49% are converted to LDL in the blood, and 1% are taken by scavenger macrophages	Transport of cholesterol to the tissue and liver. LDL requires specific LDL receptors for their removal	Transport of cholesterol from plasma to the liver. It clears cholesterol from the circulation
Enzyme involved	Lipoprotein lipase	Lipoprotein lipase	—	—	Lecithin–cholesterol acyltransferase
Cholesterol %	4	20	55	50	15
Triglyceride %	85	50	20	10	10
Protein %	1	10	20	20	45
Diameter (nm)	100–1200	30–80	25–35	18–25	5–12
Apolipoproteins Major Others	ApoB-48 A-I, A-II, C-II, C-III	ApoB-100 E, A-I, A-II, C-II, C-III	ApoB-100 E, C-II, C-III	ApoB-100 —	ApoA-I E, A-II, C-III

TABLE 2 Key enzymes involved in lipoprotein metabolism

Enzyme	Source	Location	Function	Substrate	Outcomes	Activated by	Inhibited by	Effects of deficiency
1. Lipoprotein lipase	Adipose cells Skeletal muscle cells	Endothelial cells lining blood vessels	Hydrolysis of lipids (mainly chylomicrons and VLDL)	Chylomicrons Very low density lipoproteins (VLDL)	Remnant chylomicron Intermediate-density lipoproteins (IDL)	C-II apolipo-protein present on VLDL (acts as a cofactor)	C-III apolipo-protein (acts as a cofactor)	Increased TG Progressive coronary artery disease Decreased HDL
2. Hepatic lipase	Liver Human macrophages	Liver cells Circulation	Hydrolysis of TG in IDL	IDL (Apolipo-protein B-100)	LDL (Apolipo-protein B-100) formed: 75% taken by the liver 24% taken by other tissues 1% taken by scavenger cells	Not known	Not known	Absent IDL to LDL conversion Increased risk of CA disease
3. Hormone sensitive lipase			Mobilisation of fatty acids from adipose tissue	Triacyl-glycerol, (TG)	Diacylglycerol (DAG)	Catecho-lamines (c-AMP-dependent phospho-rylation)	Insulin	Disturbed fat metabolism and energy regulation
4. Lecithin-cholesterol acyl-transferase (LCAT)		Circulation	Reversed cholesterol transport	Cholesterol transfer from lipoproteins and cells to HDL	Transfer of free cholesterol from periphery to the liver	Apolipo-protein A-I	Not known	Accumulation of free cholesterol Athero-sclerosis Fish-eye disease

Learner's reflective questions and clinical applications

- *Why is it recommended to measure serum lipids on fasting?*
  Chylomicrons (TG–rich particles) are not present in the fasted state. If the patient is not fasted, the total TG will be raised because of the presence of TG–rich chylomicrons. If the patient is fasted and TG levels are raised, it reflects increased presence of high VLDL particles.
- *Why are higher HDL concentrations associated with cardiovascular protective effects?*
  Some studies demonstrate that HDL affects the function of platelets and the haemostatic mechanisms, possibly causing a protective effect.
- *What will be the effects of lipoprotein lipase and apoprotein C–II deficiency?*
  The result is elevation of serum TG. This is because of the persistence of high concentrations of chylomicrons in the blood (the presence of chylomicrons floating like cream on the top of fasting plasma is suggestive). C–II is present on the surface of chylomicrons. It is responsible for activation of the enzyme lipoprotein lipase and it also allows chylomicrons to bind to the lipoprotein enzyme. So if the enzyme or the apolipoprotein C–II are absent ⇨ chylomicron levels are increased in blood and increased TG (the condition is not due to increased VLDL particles) ⇨ eruptive xanthomas, retinal vein thrombosis, pancreatitis, and hepatosplenomegaly.
- *What is the mechanism underlying familial hypercholesterolaemia?*
  Absence or mutation of the LDL cholesterol receptor in the liver ⇨ increased serum cholesterol. What are the consequences of this defect?
- *What is the effect of mutations in the apoprotein B-100 gene?*
  Apoprotein B-100 is present in LDL. It facilitates the binding of LDL to the LDL cholesterol receptors present in the liver. If apoprotein B-100 is absent or defective ⇨ impaired uptake of LDL by liver cells ⇨ increased serum levels of LDL cholesterol. The clinical picture is similar to familial hypercholesterolaemia. The two conditions can be differentiated by genetic tests.
- *How can we explain the pathogenesis of fatty livers in patients with excessive alcohol intake?*
  Chronic excessive alcoholic intake may cause fatty liver (steatosis) by a number of mechanisms including:
- ⇧ delivery of free fatty acids (FFA) to the liver
- ⇩ oxidation of fatty acids by mitochondria
- ⇩ transport of lipoproteins from the liver
- ⇧ lipid biosynthesis

Useful website and article to share with my group

iVillage Total Health (http://heart.health.ivillage.com/cholesterol/cholesterol.cfm). This website contains information on cholesterol, understanding the significance of high cholesterol and risk factors caused by high LDL levels in high-risk patients.

Barnard RJ. Effects of life-style modification on serum lipids. Arch Intern Med 1991; 151(7):1389–1394.

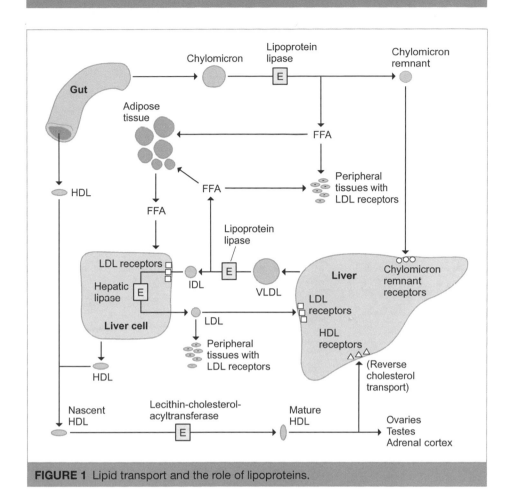

FIGURE 1 Lipid transport and the role of lipoproteins.

Appendix D

EXAMPLES OF ASSESSMENT QUESTIONS

Group 1: Multiple-choice questions (MCQs)
Group 2: Extended-matching questions (EMQs)
Group 3: Short-answer questions (SAQs)
Group 4: Problem-based learning-style (PBL) questions
Group 5: Constructed-response questions (CRQs)

GROUP 1: MULTIPLE-CHOICE QUESTIONS

Question 1

Maria Roberts is a 10-year-old primary school student on insulin for her diabetes mellitus, which was diagnosed 2 years ago. Over the last 2 days, she has complained of generalised fatigue, fever, thirst and frequent urination. She has lost her appetite, has nausea and has vomited twice. Because she is not eating, her mother has given her half her usual insulin dose. Maria is admitted to the hospital for further assessment. On examination, she appears pale, dehydrated and is hyperventilating. Examination of the cardiovascular and respiratory systems is normal. Arterial blood and urine samples are sent to the laboratory for analysis.

Which *one* of the following sets of results in the table below would you expect in her condition?

	Plasma pH (N = 7.28–7.44)	Plasma [HCO_3^-] (N = 21–28 mmol/L)	Urine pH
A	7.54	22	Alkaline
B	7.41	25	Acid
C	7.39	15	Alkaline
D	7.30	16	Acid
E	7.26	36	Acid

(*Answer is D*)

Question 2

Michael Mosepolee is a 19-year-old African student who presents to the emergency department of a local hospital with severe abdominal pain. Michael has had similar painful episodes since he was about 3 years old. On examination, he is in pain. His blood pressure is 120/80 mmHg (100/60–130/80 mmHg), his pulse is 110/min (60–100/min) and his body temperature is 36.9°C (36.6–37.2°C). His abdomen is soft and not tender and no other abnormalities are detected. The results of his full blood examinations are as follows:

      Haemoglobin (Hb): 80 g/L (Normal 115–160 g/L)
      White blood cell count (WCC): 11.5 (Normal 4.0–11.0 × 10^9/L)
      Platelet count: 350 (Normal 150–400 × 10^9/L)
Microscopic examination of peripheral blood smear is shown below.

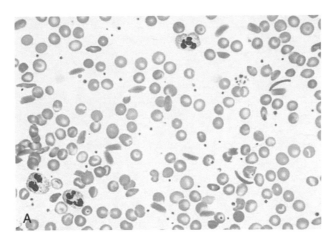

Image courtesy of Dr Robert W McKenna, Department of Pathology, University of Texas, Southwestern Medical School, Dallas, TX

1 The most likely diagnosis of Michael's presentation is:
  A. sickle cell anaemia
  B. iron deficiency anaemia
  C. alpha–thalassaemia
  D. acute appendicitis
  E. megaloblastic anaemia
(*Answer is A*)

2 Which *one* of the following investigations will help confirm your diagnosis?
  A. bone marrow biopsy
  B. abdominal X-ray
  C. haemoglobin electrophoresis
  D. serum ferritin and iron studies
  E. warm and cold antibodies
(*Answer is C*)

GROUP 2: EXTENDED-MATCHING QUESTIONS

Question 1

Theme: Drugs used in cardiovascular disorders
  A. angiotensin-converting enzyme (ACE) inhibitor (e.g. captopril)
  B. angiotensin receptor blocker
  C. spironolactone (aldosterone antagonist)
  D. beta–adrenoceptor antagonist
  E. digoxin
  F. dopamine
  G. amrinone
  H. intravenous nitroglycerin
  I. amiodarone
  J. triamterene
  K. isosorbide dinitrate
For each patient select the drug most likely to be recommended

1 A 58-year-old female presents with acute anterior myocardial infarction. Her blood pressure is 80/50 mmHg, pulse rate is 140/min, temperature 36.7°C, respiratory rate 25/min. There are bilateral crepitations on respiratory examination. Her 12-lead ECG shows no arrhythmia but changes suggestive of massive acute anterior myocardial infarction. (*Answer is F*)

2 A 49-year-old female presents with shortness of breath and signs of heart failure. Her pulse is irregularly irregular. She has been on no treatment prior to her presentation. (*Answer is I*)

3 A 58-year-old male is treated with an ACE inhibitor for heart failure following myocardial infarction. Three months later, he develops cough and investigations including chest X-ray reveal no clues for the cause of his cough. (*Answer is B*)

Question 2
Theme: Blood vessels supplying the brain
  A. right anterior cerebral artery
  B. left anterior cerebral artery
  C. right middle cerebral artery
  D. left middle cerebral artery
  E. right posterior inferior cerebellar artery
  F. left posterior inferior cerebellar artery
  G. right lenticulostriate arteries
  H. left lenticulostriate arteries
For each patient with neurological abnormalities, select the artery that is most likely to be responsible

1 A 65-year-old right-handed man presents with inability to use his right arm and leg. On examination, he has weakness of the right lower part of his face, limited voluntary dorsiflexion of the right foot, and extensor plantar response on the right side. He is unable to speak but appears to understand. (*Answer is D*)

2 A 53-year-old female presents with repeated vomiting and nausea. On examination, she has diplopia, left-sided facial weakness and difficulty to swallow (left-sided palsy of cranial nerves 9 & 10). She also has right-sided loss of pain and temperature sensations. (*Answer is F*)

GROUP 3: SHORT-ANSWER QUESTIONS

Question 1
Discuss the role of parietal cells in the secretion of hydrochloric acid (HCl) in the stomach. Briefly discuss the different mechanisms by which pharmacological agents may control HCl secreted by parietal cells.

Question 2
Briefly discuss the bone cells and their functions. Discuss the hormonal control of bone mineral metabolism. You may use flow charts to illustrate your answer.

GROUP 4: PROBLEM-BASED LEARNING-STYLE QUESTIONS

Question 1

Michael Martin, a 58-year-old worker is admitted to a Melbourne hospital because of progressive jaundice, weakness, weight-loss and mild anaemia over the last 3 months. He drinks 1–2 glasses of wine every day but he admits that he has increased his drinking since the death of his only daughter at the age of 20, about 5 months ago. On examination, Mr Martin is jaundiced. He has no spider angiomas or palmar erythema. His vital signs are normal.

Abdominal examination:

- a non-tender mass is felt below his right costal margin (most likely the gallbladder)
- no palpable spleen
- no shifting dullness
- digital rectal examination is normal
- urinalysis: bilirubin +++

Cardiovascular and respiratory examinations are normal

Investigations reveal:

Blood test	Patient	Normal range
Total bilirubin	90	0–19 µmol/L
Serum albumin	41	35–50 g/L
Aspartate aminotransferase (AST)	44	0–40 U/L
Alanine aminotransferase (ALT)	59	0–55 U/L
Gamma glutamyltransferase (GGT)	134	0–50 U/L
Alkaline phosphatase (ALP)	850	0–120 U/L

In the table below, in the first column, list the three most likely causes (hypotheses) of Mr Martin's jaundice. Your hypotheses should be consistent with the information provided in the history, examination and investigation results. For each hypothesis, write brief notes (in point form in the table), indicating the evidence for and against each hypothesis you have chosen.

Hypothesis	Evidence (Supportive)	Evidence (Against)
1.		
2.		
3.		

Question 2

Peter Roberts, a 63-year-old manager of a real estate company, comes in to see his local GP, Dr Sam Andar, because of upper abdominal pain for the last 14 hours. He says, 'The pain started last night and it was partly relieved with the ingestion of yogurt'. Further questions reveal that Mr Roberts has nausea but no vomiting and his appetite remained unchanged. He has not noticed any changes in his body weight or his bowel habits but he noticed this morning that his stools were soft and black.

Mr Roberts has smoked an average of 20 cigarettes per day for the last 30 years. He drinks 3 glasses of wine daily and about 6 or 7 on the weekends. His brother died at the age of 70 from oesophageal cancer and his father died from a heart attack. His mother died when he was young. He takes no medications but this week started to take ibuprofen, over-the-counter medication, for pains in his right knee.

His vital signs are:

Vital signs	Patient	Normal range
Blood pressure	110/70 mmHg (supine position) 90/60 mmHg (sitting position)	100/60–130/80 mmHg
Pulse rate	110/min	60–100/min
Temperature	36.9°C	36.6–37.2°C
Respiratory rate	22/min	12–16/min

Abdominal examination:
- tenderness in the epigastrium
- liver and spleen are not palpable
- rectal examination: soft black stool on the examining gloved finger

You identify abdominal pain as one of Mr Roberts' major problems. Use your knowledge of basic and clinical sciences to describe the mechanisms underlying his abdominal pain. You may use a flow chart or point form in answering this question.

GROUP 5: CONSTRUCTED-RESPONSE QUESTIONS

Michael Louise is a 25-year-old scientist who presents to his GP because of recurrent recent palpitations. He is not on any medications and does not smoke. He gives no past history of cardiovascular or respiratory disease. On examination, he looks anxious; his pulse is 130/min, blood pressure 110/70 mmHg, temperature 37°C and respiratory rate 20/min. A 12-lead ECG was done (see figure below).

Questions
A. What is your diagnosis?
B. What further information might you want to know from history questions?

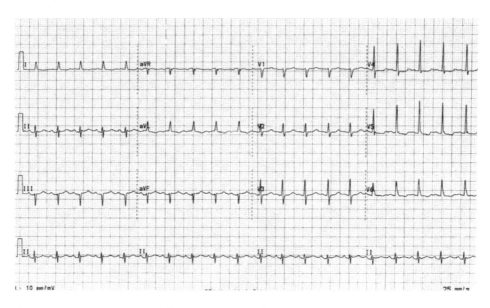

Courtesy of Professor Dr Hamed Omar, Universiti Teknologi MARA, Malaysia.

Further history questions reveal that he has had loose bowel motions for the last 3–5 months, he has noticed some tremors in his fingers and at times he drops things and always feels anxious.

C. What body systems would you like to examine? Explain your reasons.
D. What laboratory tests would you like to order for him? Explain how the results of each test will help you.
E. What are your management plan and management options?

Glossary

360-degree evaluation a mechanism for evaluating performance based on feedback from people the person comes in contact with, for example, peers, patients, nurses, clinicians, medical educators

active learning student control of their learning. Commonly used in problem-based learning and similar teaching approaches where the teacher's role is to facilitate learning rather than provide information

anatomy the science of the structure of organisms, especially of organisms such as the human body

biochemistry the chemistry of the chemical compounds and processes in organisms

bioethics study of the ethical implications of medical, biological and environmental research

biology the science of the structure, function, development and life processes of living organisms

brainstorming group discussion to produce answers to solutions and new ideas. Used in problem-based learning when the group identifies key information in the trigger, generates hypotheses and discusses available evidence. It is usually facilitated by a scribe recording on a whiteboard the key information produced by group members

CAL see computer-aided learning

case-based teaching a strategy in which cases are used to facilitate teaching. The teacher uses leading questions to direct students towards a particular response. Case-based teaching differs from problem-based learning in a number of ways. For example, in case-based teaching, cases are distributed to students at the beginning of the course, allowing students to prepare before discussing the cases as a class. The educational objectives are also given to students with each case

clinical reasoning the process of collecting information, weighing the evidence for and against each hypothesis, interpreting clinical findings, making decisions and providing justification for clinical decisions

clinical skills expertise in communication (history taking, explaining a diagnosis to a patient, telling peers about a case), medical interviewing, physical examination (observation, percussion, palpation, and auscultation), making a final diagnosis, ordering and arranging investigations, interpreting results, designating a management plan and discussing it with the patient, educating patients and their families, and following-up of patients

Cochrane Library an international, not-for-profit, independent organisation that provides clinicians, consumers and researchers with up-to-date and accurate information about the effects of healthcare. An online resource that can be used to support healthcare decisions and inform people receiving care about the best options available for their treatment. For more information see: http://www.nicsl.com.au/cochrane/guide_whatiscl.asp

cognitive skills mental skills used in the process of acquiring new knowledge. Include processes such as reasoning, generating hypotheses, searching for new information and interpreting findings

collaborative learning a method in which students work together in small groups towards a common goal

communication skills key interpersonal skills consisting of good listening skills, the ability to ask relevant questions, give constructive feedback and use body language, space, eye contact and humour to build rapport

competence being capable of performing a function. Medical competence includes patient care, medical knowledge, problem-based learning, interpersonal and communication skills, professionalism and system-based practices

computer-aided learning a teaching method that uses computers in the presentation of structural materials. Designed to enhance interaction, thinking processes and engagement of learners. Also known as 'computer-assisted instruction'

concept map the organisation of information by using networks and links to explain relationships between concepts and key information

constructed-response questions open-ended, short-answer questions used in summative and formative assessment. They measure the application of knowledge, test cognitive skills and understanding of content knowledge. A range of stimuli may be used. For example, the stem of the question may be followed by a timeline, chart, radiology film or image of an anatomical structure

continuous medical education educational activities designed to help practising medical professionals maintain, develop and increase their knowledge, skills and professional performance

cooperative learning see collaborative learning

core curriculum the central and most essential knowledge, skills, competencies and attitudes a student needs to develop during a course

critical thinking intellectually disciplined process of activities including analysis, synthesis, evaluation, application, observation, reflection, reasoning, communication, conceptualising and constructing new information. Incorporated in a number of modes of thinking such as historical, moral, philosophical and mathematical thinking

CRQs see constructed-response questions

cybermedical skills the skills needed for cybermedicine (the process of applying the internet to medical activities). Based on the use of systems such as medical informatics and computer-aided learning

decision making the competency to make decisions on the basis of evidence available from patients' symptoms, medical history, clinical examination and investigation results

deep learner a learner who keeps a balance between the big picture and fine details, reflects on what they have learnt, establishes links between what they know and new knowledge learnt. They are able to apply knowledge learnt to solve new problems and they maintain a balance between theory and practice

diagnosis identification of diseases or conditions by scientific evaluation of symptoms, medical history, clinical signs, investigation results and medical procedures

dysfunctional group in problem-based learning, groups are described as dysfunctional when they do not establish ground rules, use shortcuts in their discussion, do not use tutorial time effectively, do not dig deeper and tend to favour superficial learning, do not emphasise understanding and critical thinking, waste their time in non-productive discussions and do not know their roles or share responsibilities

EBL see evidence-based learning

EMQs see extended-matching questions

enquiry plan usually consists of open-ended questions, collection of new information, interpretation and analysis of data, drawing of conclusions, use of new information to rank hypotheses. Used to meet the PBL objective of providing students with the opportunity to aks open-ended questions to refine hypotheses.

evaluation the process of appraisal to ascertain the effectiveness of teaching and learning activities. Tools used in this process include questionnaires, surveys, focus groups, performance measurement and collaborative action research

evidence-based learning learning strategies such as sharing what is learnt with others, discussing new concepts with group members to foster deep understanding and retention of information in the long-term memory

evidence-based medicine the application of current best evidence from scientific research to medical practice, for example, the risks and benefits of a medication under certain conditions

extended-matching questions (EMQs) multiple-choice questions organised into sets using one list of options for all items in the set. EMQs test the application of knowledge and deep understanding by using 4 or 5 case scenarios to address one theme

facilitating questions open-ended questions that encourage discussion

facilitator the tutor or other staff member who oversees a problem-based learning tutorial

feedback supplying information about the result of an activity; an evaluation

formative assessment assessment designed to guide future learning, provide reassurance, promote reflection and foster learning. Takes various forms such as self- and peer assessment in tutorials, self-assessment using an online bank of questions or interactive multimedia, assignments, quizzes, mid-semester examination

histology the science of studying and identifying cells, intracellular structures and tissues through examination of specially fixed, sectioned and stained tissue under the microscope

histopathology the study of diseases at cellular and tissue levels

hybrid problem-based learning course a course that uses a mix of problem-based learning and other learning approaches

hypothesis a statement that proposes a possible explanation for a phenomenon or problem. An hypothesis needs to be tested, confirmed or excluded

immunology The study of the structure, function, immune response and diseases affecting the immune system

informatics the study of information; its structure, its communication and its use

integrated learning learning which emphasises learning across disciplines. In problem-based learning this is done by using cases

interdisciplinary education see interprofessional education

interpersonal skills these consist of communication skills (active listening and verbal skills), social skills (good eye contact, body language, ability to build rapport with others) and emotional intelligence (self-awareness, empathy and emotional maturity)

interprofessional education collaboration between medical, other healthcare professionals and providers of social services. Targets strategies to provide best-possible service to patients. Also known as: 'multiprofessional education', 'shared teaching', 'interdisciplinary education' and 'trans-disciplinary education'

learning issues in problem-based learning, the gaps in knowledge to be filled by student's own research

learning objectives objectives that highlight the learning outcomes. Should be consistent with the structure of the curriculum and should be precise

learning style the way people learn; can be classified as superficial, deep or strategic. Over time a student may use more than one approach although they have a preference for one style

life-long learning the provision and use of learning opportunities at all ages and in various contexts. It is particularly important in healthcare to keep up to date with new knowledge and changes in practice

logbook a student's record of their work, widely used in medical and other healthcare schools as an evaluation tool to assess commitment to completing tasks, certain clinical skills, how students handle challenges and the types of errors they make

MCQs see multiple-choice questions

mechanisms study of the sequence of events responsible for a change. In medical sciences, these are usually addressed at body system, organ, cellular and molecular levels

medical informatics an emerging discipline that focuses on the study, creation and implementation of electronic systems to improve communication, understanding and management of medical and healthcare information. 'The intersection of information science, computer science and health care' (Wikipedia)

mentor a trusted friend, counsellor or teacher, usually with more experience than the mentee, who offers their expertise to help the mentee in their career

MEQs see modified-essay questions

metacognitive skills learner's awareness of their own knowledge and learning skills and the skills they need to manage their own cognitive processes

microbiology the study of the biology of microorganisms such as bacteria, algae, protozoa and fungi, as well as the diseases and pathological processes caused by these microorganisms

mind map organises information by placing a main 'theme' also known as 'main items' or 'topic title' in the centre of the map while all subheads are placed on the periphery extending from, or on one side, of the centre of the map. Mind mapping produces an organised growing structure composed of keywords, key actions, changes, images and principles

mini-clinical evaluation exercise a focused, brief and observed clinical encounter followed by immediate feedback provided by the examiner. Can occur in various settings, e.g. emergency department, inpatient. Students are expected to complete 3 or 4 exercises. Each encounter is with one patient and students are expected to complete each in 15--20 minutes

modified-essay questions consist of a brief case scenario followed by two or three questions. Widely used in medical and other healthcare schools; designed to assess application of knowledge, interpretation of findings, generation of hypotheses, provision of justification

molecular biology the study of biochemical interactions and cellular processes at a molecular level

multiple-choice questions examinees are asked to select one or more of the choices from a list. Can be divided into two main groups: those that require the examinee to indicate a singe response (one best answer) and those that require the examinee to indicate all responses that are correct (true/false)

multiple-mini interview students are guided through 10 interviews, each 10 minutes long. At each interview, the candidate is presented with a brief case scenario designed to assess one of the non-cognitive skills

multiprofessional education see interprofessional education

non-cognitive skills skills or behaviours such as empathy, integrity, communication and interpersonal skills. Acquisition of such skills is part of the professional education of healthcare workers

objective structured clinical examination (OSCE) consists of a series of timed stations at which students are asked to complete a task. At some stations, students may be observed by one or two examiners while carrying out the task

online assessment the delivery of examination questions, usually multiple-choice questions, to students via online computers. Advantages are: reduction in time needed for marking, allows inclusion of images or multimedia in questions, tests can be scored immediately allowing immediate online feedback and results are easy to collect, analyse and assess

OSCE see objective structured clinical examination

passive learning learning in teacher-centred curricula; lectures are often used for the delivery of information. Fosters rote learning and memorisation rather than active participation, critical thinking, self-directed learning and construction of new information

pathology the science of disease processes as observed at body system, organ, cellular, molecular and biochemical levels

pathophysiology the study of the physical manifestations of disease and the underlying mechanisms responsible for the local and systemic changes caused by disease processes and the sequence of events underlying the disease progress

PBL see problem-based learning

pedagogy the function, work or art of teaching

peer assessment examining a peer's work and comparing it against predefined criteria agreed by group members and the faculty. Has been used in higher education for some years and been shown to enhance development of self-motivation, responsibility and reflective learning. Ground rules must be established before implementation

pharmacology the study of drugs with regard to origin, chemistry, absorption, metabolism, excretion, therapeutic effects, side-effects and contraindications

physiology the study of the biochemical and metabolic processes and functions of body systems, organs and cells

physiotherapy the study and management of congenital and acquired movement disorders through education, retraining of movement patterns, specific exercises for improving strength and motor control

portfolio collection of work that represents a student's learning, progress and achievement over time. Designed to increase self-directed learning, stimulate reflection and deep understanding and facilitate progress via feedback. Sometimes presented as an e-portfolio

problem effectiveness ability of case writers to create a well-structured case reflecting the pre-set faculty-generated learning objectives. Factors that may enhance problem effectiveness are: design of the case, flow of the case, authenticity of content, facilitating questions embedded in the case template

problem-solving learning teaching students how to solve problems. (Problem-based learning uses problems as a vehicle to drive learning.)

procedural knowledge the knowledge of how to act in a situation: the steps to follow to complete a task and the precautions to take

professionalism the willingness of doctors and healthcare professionals to subordinate their interests to meet the needs of patients and the community

reflective journal very similar to portfolios but reflective journals are less comprehensive and usually aim to develop students' self-directed learning and learning by reflection

reflective learning the use of reflective journals by students to enhance learning through critical evaluation of what is learnt, how to improve the learning process and learning from new experiences, difficult situations, challenges and mistakes

reliability a key quality for assessment tools which should be constructed in such a way that, if repeated over time, examinees will achieve similar results

rote learning memorisation of information by repetition without explanation of principles taught or justification

schema the construction of information in a meaningful way to facilitate its storage. A diagram, plan or scheme that allows organisation of related components and visualisation of relationships and interactions in a system, organ or structure

scribe in a problem-based learning setting, a scribe is the student who records on the whiteboard the information discussed by the group

self-assessment a process by which learners assess their own performance against standardised criteria

self-directed learning learners are responsible for their learning. In problem-based learning it may involve mastering self-guided research, using electronic dialogues and reflective journals, constructing new information and applying information learnt to problems presented

self-motivation the ability to reach a goal without being influenced by another person

self-regulated learning see self-directed learning

simulated patient an individual trained to act as a real patient. Their use allows medical and other healthcare students to practise and improve clinical and communication skills for an actual patient encounter

small-group learning learning in small groups of 8–10 students. Encourages student-centred approaches, collaborative learning, critical thinking and self-directed learning

strategic learning learners construct their own meanings, become aware of their own learning needs, plan their learning and target specific objectives and outcomes

student-centred in problem-based learning students control their learning: identify gaps in their knowledge, research for new information, construct the information learnt, critically assess their learning needs and apply the information learnt to solve new problems

subject guide an aid prepared by course coordinators and the faculty to help students understand the objectives of a course and manage their learning. Often in the form of an electronic document that can be downloaded from the faculty website

summative assessment assessment of the skills, knowledge and attitudes that students acquire during the semester or year. Designed to ensure that students have achieved required competencies/skills, determine their level of achievement and officially declare that they have fulfilled the requirements of a particular stage and can progress to the next stage

superficial learning the learner focuses on unrelated parts of a task, does not link theory with applications, spends insufficient time identifying evidence and arguments, memorises factual knowledge, does not apply critical thinking strategies

task-based learning learning through doing and completing tasks. In problem-based learning, tasks can include posters, logbooks, brochures, pamphlets, oral presentations, portfolios, videos, websites and research projects

tag test used in practical examinations. Items such as dissected cadavers, body organs and pathology specimens are tagged and students are asked questions related to the tagged elements

team learning see collaborative learning

telemedicine the delivery of medicine at a distance by for instance, phone, satellite technology or video-conferencing when the provider and patient are located at a distance from each other

trigger the starting point of problem-based learning cases. Usually in the form of 5 or 6 lines of text providing key information about the patient, including three or four of the presenting problems. May also include a visual trigger in the form of a single image, a series of images, a video clip, a cartoon or investigation results such as chest X-ray, pathology report or urine sample

triple-jump examination assesses students' clinical problem-solving processes and competence in self-directed learning. The three steps are (1) student reads written problem and discusses problem with the tutor. Student then selects some tasks related to the case for further learning and decides on key issues to be researched. (2) Student uses relevant resources and collects the information needed to construct new information to address the issues identified. (3) Student reports back to the tutor, presents their findings and provides a summary for the problem. The tutor provides feedback on the way in which the student addressed the problem.

tutor in problem-based learning tutorials the tutor facilitates information flow. Emphasis on the academic or clinical status of the tutor is minimised: their main task is to empower the group, facilitate the discussion and ensure the group works effectively

tutor assessment may take the form of a standardised report and is the tutor's feedback on each student in the group. Enables assessment of areas not examined by conventional methods, for example, listening skills and interaction with other members in the group, personal attributes, dealing with uncertainties, handling challenging situations and contributing to group dynamics

tutor guide in problem-based learning, it is the information provided to each tutor to improve their knowledge of the case being taught. Usually provides essential diagrams, key open-ended questions to enhance discussion and key information to ensure effective facilitation

validity a key quality for assessment tools which should be constructed in such a way that they do measure what they are intended to measure. For example, the validity of MCQs might include the extent to which a test is able to measure the subject matter, pre-identified cognitive skills and educational outcomes, and the certainty with which the test can assess students' performance

Index

continued ...

continued …

continued ...

continued …

Made in the USA
Lexington, KY
10 May 2014